T0264654

Organ Transplantation in Religious, Ethical and Social Context: No Room for Death

Organ Transplantation in Religious, Ethical and Social Context: No Room for Death

William R. DeLong, MDiv
Editor

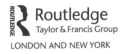

Routledge
Taylor & Francis Group

LONDON AND NEW YORK

First Published 1993 by The Haworth Press, Inc.

Published 2013 by Routledge
711 Third Avenue, New York, NY 10017 USA
2 Park Square, Milton Park, Abingdon, Oxfordshire OX14 4RN

First issued in paperback 2016

Routledge is an imprint of the Taylor and Francis Group, an informa business

Organ Transplantation in Religious, Ethical and Social Context: No Room for Death has
also been published as *Journal of Health Care Chaplaincy,* Volume 5, Numbers 1/2 1993.

© 1993 by Taylor & Francis. All rights reserved. No part of this work may be reproduced or
utilized in any form or by any means, electronic or mechanical, including photocopying, microfilm
and recording, or by any information storage and retrieval system, without permission in writing
from the publisher.

Library of Congress Cataloging-in-Publication Data

Organ transplantation in religious ethical and social context : no room for death / William R. De-
    Long, editor.
        p. cm.
    Includes bibliographical references.
    ISBN 1-56024-470-4 (acid-free paper)
    1. Transplantation of organs, tissues, etc.—Patients—Pastoral counseling of. 2. Transplanta-
tion of organs, tissues, etc.—Religious aspects. 3. Transplantation of organs, tissues, etc.—Moral and
ethical aspects. I. DeLong, William R.
RD 120.7.0723 1993
174'.25—dc20   93-29164
                                                                                                         CIP

ISBN 13: 978-1-138-97765-5 (pbk)
ISBN 13: 978-1-56024-470-7 (hbk)

Organ Transplantation in Religious, Ethical and Social Context: No Room for Death

CONTENTS

ABOUT THE EDITOR

William R. DeLong, MDiv, FCOC, is Chaplain at the University of Arizona Health Sciences Center in Tucson, where he has been chaplain to the cardiac transplant team for six years. A member of the bioethics committee for the University Medical Center, he lectures on ethics within the colleges of medicine, nursing, and psychology. Chaplain DeLong has published several papers on transplantation in medical, nursing, and pastoral care journals, including the *Journal of Pastoral Care, Transplantation, Nursing Management*, and the *Care-Giver Journal.* He is a member of the board of directors for the Arizona Organ Bank and is on the editorial staff of two professional journals.

Preface

We live in a complex world. The world of medicine completely doubles its knowledge base every two years. And, thrown into the midst of high technology and miracle cures are men and women, fathers, mothers, and children all coming because their bodies are failing, their hopes diminished, and fear abounding.

Nowhere is this more evident than in the world of organ and tissue transplantation. Here, because of some tragic and unforeseen event, some family member has decided to donate an organ or tissue so that some person, generally unknown, will live, or increase their quality of life. Here, in this world, tragedy and hope are intermingled, life and death pitted against each other, in the dramatic world of transplantation.

In this world, families are presented with the knowledge that their loved ones will only live for perhaps two years unless they want to "go the route of a transplant." In this world, health care workers see people on the edge of death undergo surgery and sometimes walk out of the hospital to return to work or some other life endeavor. In this world, families are asked in the moment of despair, tragedy, and grief, to donate the organs of their, usually young, loved one so that some surgical team from some part of the country may come in, take it, and implant it into the body of another.

In this world of transplantation, health care chaplains are asked to understand, and sometimes explain why a young person might take

[Haworth co-indexing entry note]: "Preface." DeLong, William R. Co-published simultaneously in *Journal of Health Care Chaplaincy* (The Haworth Press, Inc.) Vol. 5, No. 1/2, 1993, pp. xvii-xviii; and: *Organ Transplantation in Religious, Ethical and Social Context: No Room for Death* (ed. William R. DeLong) The Haworth Press, Inc., 1993, pp. xiii-xiv. Multiple copies of this article/chapter may be purchased from The Haworth Document Delivery Center. Call 1-800-3-HAWORTH (1-800-342-9678) between 9:00-5:00 (EST) and ask for DOCUMENT DELIVERY CENTER.

© 1993 by The Haworth Press, Inc. All rights reserved.

his own life. They are asked to understand complex medical concepts like "brain death" and explain it to a grieving father. They are asked to hope with people who have been told there is no hope. They are asked to pray with families who must let go of the hope, the miracle cure, knowing that rejection has finally taken their loved one and ended this particular journey.

Chaplains involved with transplant programs must grapple with complex ethical questions. Should they go and make an appeal to a local congregation on behalf of a thirty eight year old father, forced to fund raise because his HMO will not pay for the procedure needed to save his life. Should they confront the transplant surgeons when another candidate is being considered for transplantation when everyone knows that his drug abuse has wasted his liver? Should the surgeon stand against her emotions when a cardiac candidate is asking to have another transplant when she knows that the patient does not correctly follow his medical regime?

What are the pastoral and theological issues that arise when technology is used to extend life? What is the role of stewardship when we consider the giving of organs? What does it mean when a 68 year old man wants to have a transplant because his heart is wasted by excessive living ending in myocardial infarctions? Should we pronounce the religious belief that this life is not all there is? What does the Christian scripture mean when it says that no greater love has one than to lay down his life for another (paraphrase)?

These are some of the questions which challenge hospital chaplains in transplant centers around the world. Increasingly chaplains are being drawn into the debate which occurs in the world of transplantation. Chaplains have a unique story and perspective to bring to this debate. My hope is that in this volume, we will begin to discuss and dialogue about our role, our identity, our purpose and our function in the world of transplantation. If we are able to sharpen some of our clinical skills we will benefit our patients and staff. If we create a dialogue with which to engage surgeons, administrators, nurses and patients about the process of transplantation, then this volume has been worth the added work and pressure.

William R. DeLong, MDiv

Introduction

William R. DeLong, MDiv

Where do we begin? The world of transplantations, as you are about to read, may begin with a patient in need of surgery in order to save his or her life. It may begin with a tragic accident, leading to brain death, which makes donation of an organ possible. It may begin with the dedication and skill of surgeons, nurses, transplant coordinators, and chaplains. Since I am unable to answer this question, I simply choose to begin this volume with a section that looks at the team members who work daily with transplant patients and their families.

The transplant surgeon is the team member who leads the program. He or she, makes the choices of who is to be a candidate, who receives an organ when it becomes available, and who does not. The surgeon is the one who makes transplantation possible. What is his view of the chaplain and the chaplain's work on the transplant team. Jack Copeland, gives us his thoughts on this topic.

Tim Thorstenson, a chaplain on a transplant team, follows the surgeon's view of a chaplain by telling us what he thinks are the main ingredients for a good chaplain working with transplant patients. Tim explores the identity, role and task of the chaplain. Between these two articles, a well rounded picture is created.

Another key member of the transplant team is the transplant

[Haworth co-indexing entry note]: "Introduction." DeLong, William R. Co-published simultaneously in *Journal of Health Care Chaplaincy* (The Haworth Press, Inc.) Vol. 5, No. 1/2, 1993, pp. 1-3; and: *Organ Transplantation in Religious, Ethical and Social Context: No Room for Death* (ed. William R. De-Long) The Haworth Press, Inc., 1993, pp. 1-3. Multiple copies of this article/chapter may be purchased from The Haworth Document Delivery Center. Call 1-800-3-HAWORTH (1-800-342-9678) between 9:00-5:00 (EST) and ask for DOCUMENT DELIVERY CENTER.

© 1993 by The Haworth Press, Inc. All rights reserved.

coordinator. Anne Macdonald tells us about the special relationship of the transplant coordinator and the transplant patient. Taking us through the cardiac transplant process, Anne tells us what it is like to be in this unique position.

Clearly one role of the transplant team is to decide who will undergo transplantation when an organ becomes available. Stacie Geller and Terry Connolly question how non-medical factors influence the decision. They tell us about the role of psychosocial issues in transplant decision making.

Shifting from the role of the team members, we consider a specific group of cardiac transplant patients. Marilyn Cleavinger and Richard Smith, both engineers in the Artificial Heart Program at University Medical Center, educate us about the increasing role of technology in organ substitution. I then follow this with some of the pastoral care issues which arise when mechanical assist devices are used to keep patients alive until a compatible heart is located.

The second section of this volume looks at ethical questions which arise from transplantation and organ donation. Therese Lysaught provides food for thought as she considers the use of rites of the sick from within the Christian community and their implication for transplantation. Her perspective is unique and challenging for all concerned with caring for the sick and dying.

Art Caplan follows this article with some thoughts about scarcity and the role of religious leaders in this social dialogue. Caplan challenges the religious leaders to act instead of react as the issues of organ scarcity begin to impact the way medical science proceeds.

Close on the heels of Dr. Caplan is Deborah Mathieu, a medical ethicist in the Department of Political Science at the University of Arizona. Deborah's article invites us to consider just how far we will go in order to prolong life within the real world of scarcity.

Transplantation is considered from a catholic and interfaith perspective by Jeremiah McCarthy. He looks at some of the benefits to society by having transplantation and considers some of the moral and religious issues which arise.

The final section of the volume is dedicated to theological and pastoral perspectives concerning transplantation. Donald Capps starts the discussion by looking, as he is ought to do, at the language used in transplantation and considers some of the biblical resources which could help chaplains who work in the field of transplantation.

From Duke University Medical Center, Susan Nance and Bill Davis, look at organ donation and provide some theological insights concerning this interaction. In particular, they take on the notion of stewardship as it relates to organ donation and call it into question.

Finally, Ray Fitzgerald looks at organ and tissue donation from the light of theology. Ray uses "general attribution theory" to help him tease out some of the benefits of transplantation from a religious perspective.

TRANSPLANTATION: A TEAM APPROACH

The Chaplain's Role: A Cardiac Surgeon's View

Jack G. Copeland, MD

The chaplain is a member of the cardiac team. For me there is no doubt about this statement and it seems strange that anyone would question the concept. For over ten years, at the University of Arizona, the chaplain has played a major role in the care of patients undergoing conventional cardiac operations, heart transplants, and artificial heart-bridge-to-transplant procedures. The chaplain has been in attendance at our weekly transplant conference, discussing

Jack G. Copeland, MD, is the Michael Drummond Distinguished Professor of Cardiovascular and Thoracic Surgery and Chief of the Section for Cardio-Thoracic Surgery at the University of Arizona Health Sciences Center in Tucson, AZ.

[Haworth co-indexing entry note]: "The Chaplain's Role: A Cardiac Surgeon's View."Copeland, Jack G. Co-published simultaneously in *Journal of Health Care Chaplaincy* (The Haworth Press, Inc.) Vol. 5, No. 1/2, 1993, pp. 5-10; and: *Organ Transplantation in Religious, Ethical and Social Context: No Room for Death* (ed. William R. DeLong) The Haworth Press, Inc., 1993, pp. 5-10. Multiple copies of this article/chapter may be purchased from The Haworth Document Delivery Center. Call 1-800-3-HAWORTH (1-800-342-9678) between 9:00-5:00 (EST) and ask for DOCUMENT DELIVERY CENTER.

© 1993 by The Haworth Press, Inc. All rights reserved.

the patients who are being evaluated for transplantation, those who have just undergone transplantation, and those who are faced with the dilemmas of post-heart transplantation life and long term survival. The chaplain has been available and participated in many situations involving death, termination of life, high risk procedures and a wide variety of day-to-day less critical problems.

From my point of view, the chaplain has entered into dialog with the patient, nurses, physician and surgeon gracefully without forcing any issues with a receptiveness and sensitivity, as well as special training in psychology, which makes him a valuable contributing member of the team, as well as a personal resource for those around him. We have often requested the opinion of the chaplain on complex issues relating to the patient's perceptions, fears, behavior, social situation, family problems, or imminent death.

Perhaps the best approach to describing how a chaplain interacts in this setting is to describe typical situations in which interaction may take place. Clearly, dealing with life and death situations is the central theme.

CONVENTIONAL CARDIAC SURGERY

The patient entering into a conventional heart operation, of which coronary artery bypass and valve replacement are the most common procedures, comes with a keen awareness of his own morbidity and mortality. The situation tests him as a person to confront the facts, accept them, make a decision, and proceed with action. Typically all patients have some fear, a premonition of their own death, a feeling of helplessness, caught up in a world of medical personnel, a sterile appearing environment, and a 24 hour a day time clock which is totally foreign to normal existence. Family is very important for many of these patients. They reach out to family members, friends, and others for help. Many patients freely admit the need for help, others deny it, and this denial itself may be a useful tool in coping with a "bad" situation.

In the balance, on the patient's side, generally is a strong faith in medicine, and what it can accomplish, and in the physicians, surgeons, nurses, other personnel in the hospital, the hospital's record, and any other item which might support optimism. This is much the same psychology, although considerably more intense, than that which might be present in a prospective airline traveler when he thinks about his upcoming trip, a good record of his airlines and their flying personnel. For some, religious faith is also a great support.

A positive approach works best in the pre-operative setting, and patients respond well to plans which give them a role in the entire process. Generally, the more information they have about what will happen, the better they can cope. Simple things, like explaining the importance of deep breathing after discontinuation of ventilator support, describing the type of pain they might encounter, and how it relates to pain from other types of operations, how it will be treated and when it will subside and become insignificant, is also important. Rehabilitation concepts, dietary, physical, emotional and job rehabilitation are all things which come into focus, and they help bring a patient through this difficult time. This time is a test and a time when chaplains may be badly needed to provide patients with a non-medical positive perspective.

If all goes well with the operation the complexity of day-to-day recovery provides enough focus for the patient that anxiety, depression and fear are secondary to the practical priorities of the day. Within just a few weeks, with recovery, the test is over and perhaps in many cases, partially forgotten. The need for help and support is considerably less and the patient is nearly back to normal.

Problems and complications in the period after an operative procedure, however, have a different impact. The patient who has been sensitized pre-operatively to the possibility of failures, difficulty, death, pain, suffering, etc., may now be overwhelmed with the reality of his premonition. Depression is quite common and many patients find it difficult to maintain a positive attitude. The harder the situation, the more complicated and the more problems which occur, the deeper the depression and fear of impending death. Families and patients are tested profoundly. They question, now, the credibility of all those around them, the physicians, nurses, institution, procedure, and these questions may, in fact, just represent a deeper probing for answers than we see on the surface. In this situation a positive point of view, a strong support from all corners, including nurses, physicians, the chaplain, the family, is critical. It may make the difference between the patient being able to perform well and survive, as opposed to one who cannot perform well, and may loose strength not only physically, but also psychologically and emotionally and die.

Finally, although the numbers are quite small with modern technology, there are some who may die. In this day of high technology when prolongation of life often intersects with prolongation of death it may be difficult to tell when hope is lost from a medical and physical point of view. Indecision in the face of hopelessness and anxiety on the part of the family can cause great problems. At this point the patient is often comatose or so sick and depressed that his thoughts and feelings no longer enter into the daily dialog. They may be present in the form of a living will, or in the form of discussions with family or the cardiac team prior to decompensation. The real test at this time is the test of the strength of the family and friends. Full communication, of as much information as is known, is the best rule to follow. The family may consume a tremendous amount of the cardiac team's time. Often deep and lengthy discussions are conducted by the chaplain, the nurses, and the surgeons.

From a medical point of view, the key issue at times of severe illness is whether there is a chance for life, whether life as we know it could continue at some point in the future, or whether in fact the efforts, no matter how well meant, are prolonging suffering, misery, death of the patient and anguish of his family. There may be clear cut criteria, from a medical point of view, but in many cases there are not. Close interaction with the family is the only way to deal with decision making at this time.

THE TRANSPLANT AND ARTIFICIAL HEART PATIENT

In general, patients come for transplantation with a life expectancy or prognosis for survival of less than one year.

Those who are sick enough to need circulatory support with a mechanical device have an even grimmer outlook, and may have a prognosis of survival of days or weeks. These potential cardiac recipients generally have a greater perception of immediate risk, need to make peace, plan realistically, and call in strengths and supports. They are aware of the possibility of sudden death and they become proactive, selling themselves as good candidates for transplantation for a new heart, and hopefully a new way of life. Not all of these patients are good candidates. Many have contraindications which would make transplantation or artificial heart implantation not only risky, but so risky that they would probably survive for a shorter period of time if the intervention were taken. There is, therefore, a group who come with high expectations and leave with some element of disappointment, even after hearing the rationale for rejection as a transplant candidate.

Those who are chosen for transplantation have been placed on a waiting list. Unfortunately, the waiting period may be prolonged. In the case of outpatient waiting, a year or more may be required until the patient receives a heart. He must wait for those ahead of him on the list to have their "turns." In the case of inpatient waiting, for the more critical potential recipient, with intravenous cardiac support, the period may go for months. In either case, there is a constant feeling of anxiety, that one might be called for transplantation at any moment. Certainly there is a desire to be called and a frustration that the phone call doesn't happen. Depression is very commonly seen in these patients. Anxiety and sometimes hostility is seen in their family members. The possibility of the chaplain entering into this situation is good. Skilled professionals in the area of psychology and social work are also needed. We have found that a prophylactic approach to this situation is best. We assume that all patients are going to have significant problems, and we attempt to prevent and anticipate and forestall these if possible. Discussion, group discussion, and group therapy are ways in which these problems may be identified and unless they are identified, they may grow.

Following transplantation, a great transformation occurs. There is the patient who is converted to a new person. He is no longer an invalid. He is no longer incapacitated, he may work. He is often the focus of a good deal of attention and sometimes publicity. He has been the weakest and most dependent person in the social constellation. He may now become a provider. This is an overwhelming change in some families, one which may lead to social instability.

This recipient of a newly transplanted heart is not totally confident. He feels he cannot trust the new heart to keep him alive, to prevent sudden death, to allow him to return to activity. It is only time and trial and error that leads to confidence that then leads to the ability to return to normal function. Just as with conventional surgery, set-backs, problems, and complications test the patient and his family to question all that surrounds them.

In the setting of cardiac surgery, from the surgeon's point of view, the successes are highs and the failures are lows. Loss of life is a failure in technique, as well as the loss of a human being. From the nurses' point of view, loss of life is not only a failure of the medical profession to be able to prolong life, but also the loss of a friend, loss of a person, to whom the nurse has related in a personal way. Clearly there are great needs on the parts of these human beings, as well as patients, for strength, support, focus on the positive, and perspective in order to allow us to proceed with our daily work.

Identity, Role, and Task:
A Core Perspective
on Pastoral Care
with Cardiothoracic Transplantations

Tim Thorstenson, MDiv

Oscar Johnson was a 52 year-old farmer in a quiet rural area of southern Minnesota. When I met Oscar he was farming the land on which he had been born, and on which he had raised his own family. He was rooted in the rich tradition and heritage of basic values, a simple faith, and respect for all of life. He had a straightforward, no-nonsense outlook on life, particularly valuing family, community, and independence. It was not easy for him to enter into the evaluation phase of our transplant program. His emphysema had progressed to the point where he was no longer able to contribute to the tasks of farming, and his quality of life had diminished accordingly. Yet he was ambivalent about undergoing the evaluation,

Tim Thorstenson, MDiv, is a CPE Supervisor with the Department of Pastoral Care at Abbott Northwestern Hospital in Minneapolis, MN. Rev. Thorstenson has been Chaplain with the Cardio-Thoracic Replacement Program at Abbott since 1986.

[Haworth co-indexing entry note]: "Identity, Role, and Task: A Core Perspective on Pastoral Care with Cardiothoracic Transplantations." Thorstenson, Tim. Co-published simultaneously in *Journal of Health Care Chaplaincy* (The Haworth Press, Inc.) Vol. 5, No. 1/2, 1993, pp. 11-20; and: *Organ Transplantation in Religious, Ethical and Social Context: No Room for Death* (ed. William R. DeLong) The Haworth Press, Inc., 1993, pp. 11-20. Multiple copies of this article/chapter may be purchased from The Haworth Document Delivery Center. Call 1-800-3-HAWORTH (1-800-342-9678) between 9:00-5:00 (EST) and ask for DOCUMENT DELIVERY CENTER.

© 1993 by The Haworth Press, Inc. All rights reserved.

threatened by the loss of his independence, and clearly uncertain about stepping into the wilderness of modern high-tech health care, much less undergoing the rigors of lung transplantation.

Mr. Johnson was not atypical in his feeling of being somewhat overwhelmed, and in his tentative and guarded responses to our medical staff. He was not medically sophisticated and felt "out of his element." His life situation also posed something of a dilemma to the transplant team personnel. A lack of sophistication and his rural values tended to engender ambivalence in the staff about proceeding with the evaluation, paradoxically reflecting the ambivalence he himself was feeling. And his guarded, self-protected emotional affect tended to engender suspicion in his caregivers and questions about his level of compliance. His entry into the transplant "system" suggested his course would not be an easy one.

Upon first meeting Mr. and Mrs. Johnson, I wondered about the basic ethical principle of autonomy and its corollary, informed consent. Would we be able to honor their autonomy, or had we already violated it on some level by bringing them into this vast wilderness? Had the minimal information they received from their referring physician, and the brief video and the visit by the transplant coordinator, given rise to any meaningful level of true informed consent? Or were we just contributing to that feeling of being overwhelmed and isolated? As I listened to Mr. Johnson's story I began to get a feel for what they valued spiritually in their lives, for how they found meaning in life and for what gave them hope. As I did so I remember wondering if we were doing this man and his wife a disservice. I was aware of wanting to tell them that they would do well to go home and let life come to its natural, if shortened, conclusion, and not subject themselves to the uncertainty and suffering that I had witnessed so fully in so many previous cases.

But of course when choosing between dying and the chance for living, it is an understandable human response, and one of great value in our society, to "go for it," no matter what the risk. Over the course of the next several days, and then through several weeks of waiting back home, the Johnsons struggled with their decision. At times they felt strongly optimistic and encouraged, and at times they found themselves looking at despair as they wrestled daily with feelings of powerlessness and encroaching desperation. It is true that they may have felt powerless and desperate had they chosen not to continue with the process of transplantation, but I want to believe it would have been a qualitatively different experience. Even as I affirmed and supported their decision, I could not help but be aware of a nagging feeling deep within myself suggesting that we had seduced the Johnsons away from their basic values, away from their community, and away from feeling at all in charge of their own destinies.

This is the pastoral dilemma. To work in transplantation is to be a part of what can truly be a life-giving and miraculous process for our patients. And it can also be, paradoxically, life-denying and diminishing. The challenge is to be faithful in what for us is every bit as much a spiritual wilderness as it is for the patients to whom we minister.

The treasure we have in these "earthen vessels," according to Paul, is the Spirit of Life. The ancient peoples defined life according to the breath that came in and out of their bodies, and the Hebrews equated this breath with the Spirit of God, using the same word to define each. Literally, for them to breathe was to receive the Spirit of God, the Spirit of Life, to be alive.

When we do exercises of relaxation, imagery, and spiritual meditation, we begin by focusing on our breathing. To listen to our breath flow in and out is to clear our minds and bodies of discomforting feelings, and to take in the "spirit" of God which, according to the New Testament, brings comfort. Perhaps that can serve as a helpful paradigm for providing pastoral care to patients in the transplantation process. To bring spiritual comfort into the midst of their pain, and to help them get back within themselves in the face of that which is always drawing them away from their center, may literally be life-giving.

When Mr. Johnson inevitably deteriorated and was re-admitted to our hospital with end-stage emphysema, his anxiety was high and his ability to stay spiritually resourceful was exhausted. It was metaphorical for me when I was called by a nurse to address his feelings of panic and fear. Mr. Johnson was having a very difficult time breathing, and his saturations, according to the monitor, were in the mid 80's, a dangerously low level. For the next half hour we did relaxation and imagery exercises, and I spoke with him of his breathing being a process of receiving the spirit of God to give him comfort and quiet. It was by far our most significant and intimate interaction. Over the course of that half hour his saturation level rose to 95%. And yet I knew there was nothing that could prevent deterioration once again. Unfortunately, Mr. Johnson died 48 hours later, apart from his family, his farm, and his spiritual ground.

More and more, we are being confronted by the futility and frustration of "unsuccessful" outcomes. Last year in the United States there were over 25,000 people listed as transplant candidates, with only 4,000 donors. As programs proliferate and as our technology advances we are identifying more and more people attempting to cut up the same much more slowly expanding pie. As issues of both allocation and rationing take on greater importance in transplantation, given the above scenario, so is it becoming increasingly important that we clearly define the identity and role of the pastoral caregiver. As entering into the process of transplantation more and more becomes an experience in existential ambiguity, so is the need for the pastoral caregiver as both prophet and priest heightened. And just as it is becoming increasingly difficult to clarify ethical values and principles in transplantation, so is it difficult to identify role and task in a multidisciplinary health care delivery system for all members and participants.

Luther's perspective of "being in the world but not of the world" can be helpful in defining pastoral identity in the delivery of health care. There is both Old and New Testament precedent for such a view, where people of faith are referred to as "strangers and sojourners," conveying the sense that we speak from a unique and important perspective that may run counter to the way of the world. It is a difficult line to walk, both with medical staff and with patients–to serve both as a representative of the transplant team and as a corrective to what it embodies. Walking that line perhaps involves redefining the concept of stewardship. Stewardship as an ethical value involves responsibility, accountability, and commitment to one another, as well as to the principle of justice. We might say that we are called to be stewards of the process, where our identity is shaped by our responsibility and commitment to both health care professionals and to patients, where we are accountable to the values that shape our heritage. As stewards we will engage in the process of truth-telling to help clarify the values of the patient and to facilitate a process of appropriate, informed decision-making.

This necessarily involves the need to talk about death as a distinct possibility. Seventy million people die each year. We have unfortunately denied this reality by seeing death not as a process of life, framed by traditions of faith, but as a failure. We put a rouge on death. As stewards of life, we need to embrace with our patients the reality that death is a part of living. Even as we value extending life, so do we, as strangers and sojourners, embrace death as a vehicle of God's redemptive activity. To hold up such a perspective to the health care community is to facilitate justice, sustainability, and fuller participation by the physician with the patient, while decreasing the likelihood of running unnecessary and desperate risks, which may ultimately lead to increased suffering. To hold up such a perspective to the patient is to deepen compassion, solidarity, and the potential for true, intimate reflection. And to stand as an active participant in the *process* of evaluation and reflection is to sharpen our own identities as stewards of grace.

To more fully refine and define the role of the pastoral caregiver, it is important to understand the dynamics of what we might call "the abyss of high-tech/high-touch medicine," since we would do well to move from a stance of "paternalism" to a stance of "solidarity." Paternalism is the unfortunately common dynamic suggesting that we, the medical professionals, know better than the patient what is in his or her best interest. In the fast-paced and short-term world of modern diagnostic medicine, it is a seductive dynamic allowing us to rely on our experience and a diagnostic/prognostic model where human values are not directly assessed, rather than listen to and reflect with the patient.

This dynamic is borne out over and over in organ transplantation. The patient generally does not have an informed understanding of the rigors of maintenance and treatment, and so looks to professional staff for information and guidance. This automatically creates a hierarchical structure where patients see the professional as "all knowing" and themselves as dependent. Too often the medical professional fosters that dynamic and continues the experience of powerlessness by telling the patient what he or she needs to do rather than sorting through feelings and responses. This is why we put so much emphasis on the quality of "compliance" in modern health care. In the paternalistic view, there is a high value placed on the patient's compliance (that is, the ability to follow direction) rather than on integration, which I would understand as the ability to gather information and make informed medical decisions. While it is important that the patient comply with medical direction, it is also important that patients weigh the risks and benefits and sort them through with caregivers and loved ones, so that they can take "ownership" of the process and move ahead with self-esteem intact and with a sense of empowerment. When we over-emphasize compliance we fail to discern the patient's emotional and spiritual orientation and we preclude personal growth and the potential serenity that comes with acceptance and reflective integration. The patient gets "stuck" on feelings, oftentimes in fact experiencing a growing sense of frustration or powerlessness.

We see the effects of paternalism most clearly in what might be called "the gatekeeping effect," where patients find themselves wanting to please the caregiver to ensure that they will be accepted onto the transplant list and liked by the people who hold power over them regarding decision-making, such as physicians and nurses, thereby ensuring that they will be treated with favor and not run the risk that they will be discriminated against. Due to the gatekeeping effect, the patient will oftentimes withhold ambivalent feelings and not fully disclose emotional and spiritual struggles that normally accompany the disease process. The effect of this is to minimize the intimate reflection with caregivers that is so necessary for coming to terms with the painful realities of transplantation. The patient ends up feeling more isolated, not less, and the staff is lulled into believing that the effects of its paternalistic style are beneficial to the patient. As if in collusion around these dynamics, patient and staff together are unwittingly seduced into putting their trust into a potentially beneficial but still illusory vision, shaped by what has become the most technically advanced medical practice and technology of our time. And the effects of modern medicine's current high-tech/high-touch style can become, at its worst, alienating and numbing. Just as the high-tech machines and medicines that we offer are designed to provide deepened optimism and security, so is the high-touch emphasis designed to sooth and muffle patients' fears and concerns. Too often, however, we are enticed into offering high-touch paternalism, cloaked in religious authority, all in a half-hearted attempt to facilitate accommodation and compliance in the patient, defeating the true goals of pastoral care.

Against this scenario, the role of the chaplain is to become a truth-teller. I have come to deeply appreciate the tradition that sees the pastoral caregiver as having three dimensions: that of priest, prophet, and poet. We are intimately familiar with the priestly role and tend to do that quite well. To be prophet, however, means to serve as a corrective to the paternalistic tendencies of modern tertiary care while drawing our authority from within the system, by virtue of our knowledge and understanding, both of medicine and of human dynamics. To be a prophet in transplantation is to counter the gate-keeping effect by inviting patients into an intimate dialogue around their deepest fears and concerns. It is not to just walk with them through the wilderness of transplantation, but to facilitate a process of self-discovery and acceptance that necessarily involves the gathering of information and the clarifying of medical options. It is to help patients find their voice and claim their own autonomy, helping them to exercise greater rather than less responsibility for their well-being and potential outcome.

It is not uncommon for a patient to experience feelings of disorientation and powerlessness even after receiving a transplant, failing to "own" their new medical regimen, or failing to take responsibility for their recovery by maintaining a strict daily medication schedule. I have worked with a number of patients who have experienced rejection episodes as a result of being lax in their medication routines. My fear is that the failure to take full responsibility was engendered early on in their evaluation and waiting phase and that, in each case, the patient failed to engage his or her feelings at a deep level, move through resistance to an authentic level of acceptance, and integrate the changes into a life of expectation and hope. By "holding up the mirror" to the patient in a compassionate invitation to self-discovery, the chaplain facilitates a movement away from compliance and toward spiritual groundedness in an uncertain world.

To be priest and prophet in a world of high-tech medicine, where we can extend dying artificially and prolong suffering unwittingly, where we overwhelm the patient with a multiplicity of staff and physicians, and where we draw patients away from their deepest selves, the chaplain's role becomes one of helping each patient find meaning amidst the wilderness experience, re-valuing life.

Might we also see ourselves as interpreters, as ones who provide a language and a spiritual vantage point from which to explore the deeply human questions that arise when life becomes tenuous? The alienation of disease and of becoming slaves to technology entices us into silence. In deference to Douglas John Hall, it is the poet's task to speak for those who cannot; yet to facilitate the integration and acceptance that incorporates the strains of life in consciousness and facilitates an expression of feeling that brings about serenity and security. Put another way, the poet's task truly is to work to keep body and soul together, to enter into a relationship with the patient not to resolve the pain of the patient's existential experience but to help the patient live with the experience creatively and faithfully.

To facilitate the process of self-discovery and of coming to terms with an uncertain world, the necessary first task for the pastoral caregiver is to do an in-depth spiritual assessment. Such an assessment provides a vehicle for "joining with" the patient considering transplantation, and helps determine appropriate interventions with patient, family, and also with medical staff. The spiritual assessment is a process of moving into the patient's inner being to discern how the patient orders his or her world and to understand what gives meaning to his or her life. It is to determine, through the establishment of a caring professional relationship, how each patient is responding to his or her current medical reality and its accompanying life changes. There is considerable literature available to help the chaplain define the spiritual categories that are to be addressed, including levels of shame/belovedness and alienation/reconciliation, which I consider core issues. The goal of such an assessment is to understand the patient's current behaviors and expressions by evaluating with the patient his or her values and belief systems, coping mechanisms and resources, and concepts of transcendence, hope, and faith. If we are to take seriously our role as consultants in a wholistic approach to health care, then our task is to assess and diagnose spiritual issues alongside of medical diagnosis of physical needs. To help our patients bring to consciousness what holds meaning for them in the face of their crises is to empower and equip them to adjust accordingly; that is, to give them the potential to develop a deepening sense of serenity in the face of anxiety-producing stimuli.

For many if not most of our patients, the current diagnosis and unfolding prognosis confronts them with the limits of life and with their own mortality, breaking down the denial that insulates them from the terror of life. I believe this to be the universal human response in transplantation. Spiritual care begins when we acknowledge that change in orientation in our patients. To do so is to "walk into their wilderness" with them, and to "wonder" with them about the significance such change has for their lives. It is to help them explore their deeper feelings and discern that which has the "feel of truth" about it. In so doing we begin to work with the patient to help distinguish between mere optimism and a deeper level of hope, whereby each begins to access and identify unfolding spiritual values. We might say that the prescription we offer for their diagnosis and treatment is one of spiritual reflection, with the goal being one of acceptance and serenity. Far from being a paternalistic voice encouraging them to "hang on" or to "be more compliant," ours is a voice that invites them to "let go" and develop a deeper sense of trust and acceptance.

Our patients are our patients for life. They realize that it is only reasonable to expect up to ten years of life post-transplant, and that they will be lives filled with routine and not-so-routine interventions. We must begin our task of pastoral care with a spiritual assessment. As we seek to engender faithfulness in our patients to the promises of God's caring presence no matter what life has in store, so do we need to remain faithful in our commitment to our patients and to the goals of spiritual growth. It is a parallel process. Just as we ask our patients to let go of the outcome in hopes of establishing a deepened sense of trust and hope, so do we need to let go of the outcome of our spiritual interventions. When being daily confronted with the limits of medical and spiritual care, we need to be clear about our identity, role, and task, so that we can live with a healthy perspective that will free us to walk with our patients as the need arises. Our goal, then, is not to put our energies toward seeing to it that our patients survive and live through and beyond their transplants, but that they live, while they are yet alive, with decreased anxiety and deepened serenity, with an improved sense of direction and purpose, and with a heightened sense of "connectedness" with themselves, with their loved ones, and with God. To do that is to embrace our identity as "strangers and aliens," as ones who are both a part of the system and a corrective to it, as ones who are priests, prophets, and poets.

The Heart Transplant Recipient-Coordinator Relationship: Reactions to the Transplant Process

Anne Nicholson Macdonald, RN, MS

Since the first human heart transplant in 1967, heart transplantation has evolved from an experimental procedure to a therapeutic treatment modality for end-stage heart disease. In the early years the focus was primarily on patient survival, made difficult by high rates of infection and rejection. Patient survival has dramatically improved, thanks to enhanced diagnosis and treatment of rejection and infection, immunosuppressive therapy and improved donor and recipient selection criteria (Macdonald, 1990; Copeland, 1987). But while the physical complications have become less difficult to manage, psychosocial and ethical considerations have been receiving more attention.

The role of the professional clinical transplant coordinator has evolved and formalized with the rapid changes in the field of heart transplantation. The transplant coordinator role has significantly contributed to the success of heart transplantation today (Davis,

Anne Nicholson Macdonald is a Transplant Coordinator with the Department of Surgery at the University of Arizona, Tucson, AZ.

[Haworth co-indexing entry note]: "The Heart Transplant Recipient-Coordinator Relationship: Reactions to the Transplant Process." Macdonald, Anne Nicholson. Co-published simultaneously in *Journal of Health Care Chaplaincy* (The Haworth Press, Inc.) Vol. 5, No. 1/2, 1993, pp. 21-31; and: *Organ Transplantation in Religious, Ethical and Social Context: No Room for Death* (ed. William R. DeLong) The Haworth Press, Inc., 1993, pp. 21-31. Multiple copies of this article/chapter may be purchased from The Haworth Document Delivery Center. Call 1-800-3-HAWORTH (1-800-342-9678) between 9:00-5:00 (EST) and ask for DOCUMENT DELIVERY CENTER.

© 1993 by The Haworth Press, Inc. All rights reserved.

1987). The coordinator is the cornerstone of the care of the transplant patient, and is the communication link between the transplant team, ancillary services, referring physician and the recipient.

The recipient-coordinator relationship is unique and long-term in nature. The coordinator is one of the few health care professionals that is a care-giver throughout the transplant process, from the time of evaluation until death. Thus, with a positive outcome, the coordinator provides continuity of care from evaluation through transplantation and long-term follow-up.

The transplant coordinator is primarily a health care provider, with the goal of providing holistic care to meet the patient's physical and psychosocial needs. The coordinator becomes the patient's advocate, at times the "voice" of the patient, communicating his or her desires to the transplant team. The role of the coordinator is also one of facilitator, with responsibilities ranging from ensuring that the evaluation tests are completed to monitoring the patient's health post-operatively. Finally, the coordinator educates the patient regarding specifics of the transplant process, including potential complications, medical follow-up, quality of life after transplant and, perhaps most importantly, the patient's own health care monitoring.

The coordinator-recipient relationship is affected by the intensity and length of the relationship. When an intense relationship occurs, even short term, such as when the patient dies during the waiting period, the situation can be highly emotional for the coordinator. The length of the patient's survival after transplant directly impacts on the degree of loss felt by the coordinator at the time of the recipient's death. As with all relationships, time and experiences can deepen feelings of loss for the coordinator, especially if a strong bond exists between the coordinator and patient, as well as their families.

There are five significant psychological adjustment stages associated with heart transplantation: Evaluation period; Waiting period; Immediate post-operative period (hospitalization); First three months; and Long-term follow-up. These adjustment stages are similar to those initially described by Allender et al., but have been expanded (Macdonald, 1990; Allender et al., 1983).

Patients referred for transplant evaluation have end-stage cardiac disease, with a prognosis of less than 12 months survival. Generally, no other surgical or medical option exists for these patients, and transplantation is their only hope for survival. The transplant candidate and family undergo a rigorous physical and psychosocial evaluation. The evaluation is performed using a multidisciplinary team approach. The evaluation period is also an opportunity for the candidate and family to evaluate the transplant team and program.

During the evaluation period, predominant subjective emotions are anxiety and depression, in addition to ambivalence, anger, suspicion, and confusion, all complicated by mood swings. (Kuhn et al., 1990). Other common emotions are feelings of helplessness, fear, loss of control and "being in limbo." Generally, by the time a patient is referred for transplant he or she and the family understand the severity of the condition. The evaluation period, however, clearly forces the patient and family to examine their feelings regarding the potential risk and benefits of transplantation. It is important for the patient to resolve feelings of ambivalence before pursuing transplantation. Most patients, however, "prefer the uncertainty of transplantation to the certainty of death," (Christopherson, L. 1976).

Common feelings for the coordinator during the evaluation period include empathy, frustration, guilt and ambivalence. It is common to feel empathy for patients and their families, since without transplantation the prognosis is grim. Most patients place a great deal of hope in their acceptance as a transplant candidate. This can place pressure and guilt on the transplant team to feel they should accept the patient.

The coordinator provides the majority of information regarding test results to the patient. Negative test results or the patient's rejection for transplantation can be difficult to convey to the patient. In most programs, the transplant physician will "officially" refuse the patient for transplant; however, the coordinator is left to provide emotional support for the patient and family. It is hard not to feel guilty about a patient's refusal, even when transplantation would inflict additional suffering on that patient. The patient usually does not understand or believe statistics, past experience or ethical issues, not when faced with losing the last hope for long-term survival. If the patient is accepted as a marginal candidate, either physically or psychosocially, it can cause frustration or ambivalence when there are so many "good" candidates already waiting.

Once accepted for transplant, the patient enters the waiting period. This period is commonly described as "life on hold" or "waiting to live or waiting to die" (Macdonald, 1990), and is probably the most stressful period for the patient and family. The stress is worsened by the severe donor shortage. There are currently 2,268 patients waiting for cardiac transplantation in the United States alone. The majority of patients wait more than 6-12 months (UNOS, 1992). Approximately 20% of patients will die while awaiting transplantation.

The predominate emotion for the candidate during the waiting period is anxiety (Kuhn et al., 1990). Patients and their families may also experience feelings of powerlessness, competitiveness, frustration, hostility, decreased self-esteem and depression. During the waiting period, patients must balance the constant reality of their precarious health and the possibility of death, while maintaining hope for a transplant and prolonged survival. If the patient has strong religious beliefs, often death is not feared; then the patient is able to prepare for death while maintaining hope, understanding his or her fate is in God's control.

During the waiting period, family members exhibit heightened vigilance of the patient (with disregard to their own needs), protective behaviors and role reversal. This process, labeled "immersion," has been described by Mishel and Murdaugh in an exploratory study examining family adjustment to heart transplantation (Mishel M., and Murdaugh, C., 1987).

As the waiting time for a donor heart increases, it is not unusual for the transplant team, including the coordinator, to begin avoiding the patient and family. Avoidance results from frustration and guilt due to the lack of a donor heart, and the inability to change the situation (Levenson, J. and Olbrisch, M., 1987). Patients can also become obsessive about their situation, making the coordinator feel uncomfortable. Patients may exhibit "gallows humor" or the "rainy day syndrome," dwelling on or fantasizing about the death of a potential donor (Kuhn, W., Davis, M., Lippmann, S., 1988; Levenson, J., Olbrisch, M., 1987). This often results then in feelings of guilt by the patient.

Patients may become depressed, demanding and angry, as the stress of waiting increases. While decreasing contact can further aggravate the situation, it is often difficult and emotionally draining to spend time with these patients. In addition, as patients develop support networks among themselves, they often feel entitled to information about fellow patients that violates confidentiality issues for the coordinator.

There exits a "transplant window" for transplant candidates, which refers to the period of time they are an acceptable candidate, both physically and psychologically. Due to the natural progression of the patient's disease process, the patient may become too ill to undergo transplant. This can be heartbreaking, not only for the patient and family but the coordinator as well.

Death while waiting is difficult to accept. There is a feeling that the patient (and coordinator) were so close and had worked so hard for a second chance that they shouldn't have been denied. Feelings of grief are intensified if the patient had waited a particularly long time and close bonding occurred.

CASE HISTORY I

B.C., a 40 year-old single mother of three children became critically ill over a two-three week period after a viral illness causing viral cardiomyopathy. She was initially placed on an artificial heart as a bridge to transplant. Within four days she received a heart transplant; however, two days later she suffered a hyperacute rejection and was again placed on an artificial heart. She then spent eight months on a Jarvik artificial heart in the intensive care unit awaiting transplant.

During this time she suffered multiple life-threatening complications and associated painful procedures. Since she was relatively immobilized, we had many long talks during her hospitalization. Throughout that time, she demonstrated tremendous courage and a strong will to live. At times, however, she did feel frustrated and angry, describing her life tethered to the artificial heart drive system as "being a dog on a leash." She also had intervals of depression, and at one point fantasized about cutting the drive lines that powered the artificial heart.

Even though her life was intensely precarious she maintained strong faith in God's love and protection. Much of the reason she maintained a generally positive outlook was for and because of her young children. She often expressed appreciation for the extra time she was able to spend with them.

B.C. became my friend during this long hospitalization. Her quiet faith and courage were moving. While dealing with the constant potential for death, she remained hopeful of a successful transplant until her death. She died in the operating room, immediately after receiving her second transplant.

Once the transplant occurs, most patients and their families feel tremendous relief and may even be euphoric (Kuhn, W., Davis, M., and Lippman, S., 1988). These feelings are usually countered within several days by the reality and hard work of recovery. Initial euphoric feelings may be replaced with labile emotions, including depression. Emotions are intensified by the medications given, particularly steroids. During the immediate post-operative period, focus for the patient and family is centered on physical recovery. Patients begin an intensive education program, learning their medications, dietary management, cardiac rehabilitation and health care monitoring.

As the patient's physical recovery progresses, the patient and family may become fearful of potential complications, primarily rejection and infection. In addition, patients begin the process of accepting their new heart. They may experience many emotions, including guilt, regarding the death of their donor. The patient may grieve for the donor and donor family. They may also wonder about characteristics of the donor and if these characteristics can be imparted to them.

During the immediate post-operative period the coordinator focuses on monitoring the patient's progress and educating the patient and family. There is a sense of relief that the patient survived to get the transplant, alongside the understanding that the patient faces a new set of challenges. Transplantation has been commonly described as "trading one set of problems for another." The education provided by the coordinator and the level of knowledge gained by the patient is crucial to the patient's long-term survival. The coordinator feels responsible for providing a solid foundation of knowledge to equip the patient for future problems.

In the first three months post-transplant, the primary medical risk factors are infection and acute rejection. While infection and acute rejection remain a threat throughout the patient's life, the incidence decreases after three months. Complications resulting in death have decreased during the first three months; however, they may still occur. It is these complications that the patient and coordinator fear, even if that fear remains unspoken. This is perhaps the most difficult time to lose a patient, during the end of the acute phase of the transplant process, after so many challenges have already been overcome.

CASE HISTORY II

B.A., a 60 year old married man, had multiple complications, including multiple infection and rejection episodes, after his transplant. He was hospitalized the majority of the post-transplant period. Finally, during his last hospitalization, he was diagnosed with Aspergillus pneumonia, a serious, often fatal infection.

To combat his uncertainty, he attempted to maintain as much control of his situation as possible. He was intellectually involved in his care, asking questions and attempting to make sense of his myriad set of problems. He kept carefully detailed lists, grafts, and notes of all the events affecting him. At first, I found B.A.'s intense desire for detail frustrating. I soon realized, however, that by B.A. understanding our thoughts and treatment plan he was able to maintain a positive attitude and courageously battle each new complication. B.A. was also fortunate to have a loving and supportive family.

At the end of B.A.'s life, his condition had deteriorated to the point where he was maintained on a ventilator, with multiple blood pressure supporting medications and had severe brain injury. Knowing B.A.'s wishes, the family elected to withdraw support after having several meetings with the surgeon, chaplain, social worker and myself. Immediately, prior to removing B.A. from his life-supporting machines, his wife expressed her appreciation for the transplant team's effort in her husband's care. She said that she and B.A. had viewed the transplant process as an "adventure" and that they had had a very special last few months together, despite B.A.'s complications. B.A.'s family was able to spend time saying goodbye to him and prayed with the chaplain together at the bedside before his death.

In the first several months after transplant, even with a positive outcome, the patient and family are often insecure with the new identity as a transplant recipient. This insecurity is exhibited by dependence on the transplant team, usually through the coordinator. The coordinator uses this time as a weaning process, encouraging the patient to shift from reliance on the transplant team back to self and family. A primary goal for the coordinator is to promote self-care with optimal health monitoring skills and knowledge in the patient.

This period of time is described by Mishel and Murdaugh as "passage." The patient and family vacillate between feeling life will return to normal and realizing the potential for complications. Finally, the patient and family come to the understanding that the patient is vulnerable and that life has changed (Mishel, M. and Murdaugh, C., 1987).

Transplant recipients feel they are special people. They have "beaten the odds" and are joyful at being given a second chance. Most patients acknowledge their unique experience–having been near death and suddenly restored to health so fully. These feelings are often intense during the first three months. Despite the many patients that have expressed their appreciation at having a second chance, each time I am awed by God's gift of life. An example of this was a patient, hospitalized with serious complications postoperatively, who was allowed to spend some time sitting outside the hospital. After he returned to his hospital room, he said, "I just sat outside and watched the cars go by and I was happy just to be able to do that. I'm just so happy to be alive."

Alter approximately two to three months, the recipient and family return home to resume their (perhaps redefined) "normal" life. Life after transplant, however, poses significant obstacles for the recipient and family. These problems include the potential for medical complications and side-effects of the immunosuppressive medications; employment and financial stressors; family and marital strain. They add unavoidable uncertainty to the recipient and family's life.

Acute rejection and infection can occur at any time post-transplant. The complication affecting long-term survival, however, is chronic rejection or graft atherosclerosis. Graft atherosclerosis, a form of accelerated coronary artery disease, has been reported to be as high as 40-50% at five years (Pahl, E., Fricker, J., Armitage, J. et al., 1990). The diffuse nature of the disease generally necessitates re-transplantation or results in death. A cardiac catheterization is performed on a yearly basis to diagnose graft atherosclerosis. The yearly follow-up examination forces patients to consciously face their uncertain futures. Patients anxiously await the results of their catheterization. I dread reading the catheterization results with patients I am particularly fond of, especially as the years progress. It is painful to have to give them negative results.

CASE HISTORY III

S.M., a 34 year old male, was transplanted eight years earlier for idiopathic cardiomyopathy. At the time of his first transplant he was single. Since his transplant he has married and has had two children. Prior to his last hospitalization, he had been experiencing significant shortness of breath and a decreased exercise tolerance for approximately three months. After a full cardiac evaluation, he was found to have a severe restrictive cardiomyopathy.

The transplant surgeon and I met with he and his wife to discuss the only viable option for him, which is re-transplantation. S.M. is young and feels that with his family he has a great deal to live for. He underwent transplant re-evaluation and was found to be a good candidate. He is currently awaiting re-transplantation.

S.M. is an example of a patient I have grown particularly fond of over the years. I have seen him mature as a person and as a transplant recipient. He has maximized his time since his first transplant. It has been a pleasure to work with him. I was saddened with his new cardiac dysfunction and now am hopeful that he will live to receive a second transplant.

The transplant coordinator becomes an integral part of the patient's life, having been with the patient through multiple stressful periods. A bonding and caring relationship occurs. In some cases, a friendship may also develop. Transplant recipients place their trust (thus their life) in the transplant team's judgment and decisions. This trust is clearly and continually communicated, from the patient to the coordinator, throughout the transplant process. It is not unusual, then, to feel protective and responsible for the transplant recipient's well-being. Thus, when a recipient dies, perhaps many years post-transplant, it is a significant loss, not only for the family but for the coordinator and transplant team as well.

The follow-up period, the rest of the patient's life, is ultimately the most important time for the patient. This final period, labeled "negotiation" by Mishel and Murdaugh, is significant for role realignment with integration of the recipient's vulnerability and unpredictable future (Mishel, M. and Murdaugh, C, 1987). It is a continual process of growth.

It is gratifying when a patient is able to resume the activities he or she enjoys, integrating the identity as a transplant recipient with a new lifestyle. When transplantation results in an integrated recipient and family that are glad they accepted the challenge of transplantation, it makes my job as a coordinator meaningful and worthwhile. Transplantation offers a unique opportunity for a long and rewarding relationship between the transplant recipient and coordinator. Transplant recipients are special people. Their courage and spirit is inspiring and provides the foundation for the advancement of cardiac transplantation.

REFERENCES

Allender, J., Shisslak, C., Kaszniak, A., and Copeland, J. (1983). Stages of Psychological Adjustment Associated with Heart Transplantation. *Heart Transplantation*, 2(3): 228-231.

Christopherson, L. (1976). Cardiac Transplant: Preparation for Dying or for Living. *Health and Social Work*, 1(1): 58-72.

Copeland, J.G., Emery, R., Levinson, M., Icenogle, T., Carrier, M., Ott, R., Copeland, J.A., Rhenman, M., and Nicholson, S. (1987). Selection of Patients for Cardiac Transplantation. *Circulation*, 75(1): 2-9.

Davis, F. (1987). Coordination of Cardiac Transplantation: Patient Processing and Donor Organ Procurement. *Circulation*, 75(1): 29-39.

Kuhn, W., Brennan, F., Lacefield, P., Brohm, J., Sketon, V., Gray, L. (1990). Psychiatric Distress During Stages of the Heart Transplant Protocol. *The Journal of Heart Transplantation*, 9(1): 25-29.

Kuhn, W., Davis, M., and Lippman, S. (1988). Emotional Adjustment to Cardiac Transplantation. *General Hospital Psychiatry,* 10: 108-113.

Levenson, J., and Olbrisch, M., (1987). Shortage of Donor Organs and Long Waits. *Psychosomatics,* 28(8): 399-403.

Macdonald, S.N. (1990). Heart Transplantation, in Smith, S. (ed). Tissue and Organ Transplantation: *Implications for Professional Nursing Practice,* (pt 1) pp 210-23. St. Louis: CV Mosby.

Mishel, M. and Murdaugh, C. (1987). Family Adjustment to Heart Transplantation: Redesigning the Dream. *Nursing Research,* 36 (6): 332-38.

Pahl, P., Fricker, J., Armitage, J., Griffith, B., Taylor, S., Uretsky B., Beerman, L., and Zuberbuhler, J. (1990). Coronary Arteriosclerosis in Pediatric Heart Transplant Survivors. *The Journal of Pediatrics,* 116 (2): 177-183.

UNOS Statistics–Patients Waiting for Transplants (1992). National Organ Procurement and Transplantation Network, *UNOS Update,* 8(1): 18.

The Influence of Psychosocial Factors in the Heart Transplantation Decision Process

Stacie E. Geller, MA
Terry Connolly, PhD

INTRODUCTION

Over the past twenty-five years, cardiac transplantation has evolved from an experimental procedure to a well accepted therapeutic technique for end-stage heart disease. Since the early days of transplantation, many aspects of the procedure, primarily immunosuppressant therapies, have undergone continued development, with significant improvements in patient survival, rehabilitation, and quality of life (Futterman, 1988). This has resulted in a dramatic growth in both the number of cardiac transplantations and trans-

Stacie Geller is a PhD candidate at the University of Arizona in the Department of Management and Public Policy, BPA. Terry Connolly is Professor and Decision Theorist in the same department at the University of Arizona.

Address correspondence to either author at: Department of Management and Policy, BPA, University of Arizona, Tucson, AZ 85721, E-mail: connolly @ccit.arizona.edu.

[Haworth co-indexing entry note]: "The Influence of Psychosocial Factors in the Heart Transplantation Decision Process." Geller, Stacie E., and Terry Connolly. Co-published simultaneously in *Journal of Health Care Chaplaincy* (The Haworth Press, Inc.) Vol. 5, No. 1/2, 1993, pp. 33-43; and: *Organ Transplantation in Religious, Ethical and Social Context: No Room for Death* (ed. William R. DeLong) The Haworth Press, Inc., 1993, pp. 33-43. Multiple copies of this article/ chapter may be purchased from The Haworth Document Delivery Center. Call 1-800-3-HAWORTH (1-800-342-9678) between 9:00-5:00 (EST) and ask for DOCUMENT DELIVERY CENTER.

© 1993 by The Haworth Press, Inc. All rights reserved.

plant centers since the mid-1980s. In 1991, more than 2,125 cardiac transplantations were performed in the United States in more than 157 different centers (Cate & Laudicina, 1991).

The further growth of cardiac transplantation is constrained by severe organ scarcity. Estimates are that between 15,000 and 34,500 patients per year, in the United States alone, could potentially benefit from heart transplantation (Evans & Yagi, 1987; Freidman, Ozminkowski and Taylor, 1992). Recent estimates of the potential recipient population have increased, in part, because of an upward shift in the age distribution of current recipients and liberalized selection criteria. With numbers of potential recipients growing, it appears quite unlikely that the shortage of available donor hearts will be overcome. Even doubling or tripling the number of hearts currently available for transplantation would not meet demand, and increased numbers of patients are being considered for transplantation each year (Evans, 1986).

The continuing shortage of donor hearts makes selection of recipients a difficult and potentially controversial process. Roger Evans, lead author of the national heart transplantation study (1985) states that ". . . patient selection will be a constant problem associated with heart transplantation. Bluntly stated, the problem is one of deciding who will benefit when not all can." Heart transplantation, therefore, necessarily involves allocation of a scarce resource resulting in the need for selection criteria and a screening process.

In this paper we discuss the nature of patient selection criteria for heart transplantation as they currently exist, the psychosocial screening and candidate selection process in one successful heart transplantation program, and directions for future research.

PATIENT SELECTION CRITERIA

At present, the decision to accept a patient for transplant is "guided" by standard criteria formulated by the Federal Registry and generally agreed upon by the clinical specialists involved in heart transplantation. These selection criteria are a mix of medical, financial, and psychosocial considerations, with primary emphasis on medical factors. Broadly stated, the criteria are intended to maximize the probability that the recipient will survive and adapt successfully to the transplant.

Medical criteria dominate the selection process. Patients who request transplants are first evaluated to determine if they can benefit from other treatments. An assessment is made of their prognosis for survival without the transplant. A balance must be made between patients who are judged "too sick" and those judged "not sick enough." The selection of patients who are "too sick" for transplantation is a disservice both to the patient and to others on the waiting list. For the very sick recipient, survival prospects are poor; and, of course, transplanting one patient means not transplanting another. Conversely, premature transplantation of patients who are doing well on medical therapy must be avoided (Dec, Semigran, & Vlahakes, 1991).

Transplant teams in a recent GAO study (GAO, 1989) reported using relatively standard medical criteria to determine eligibility. There is general agreement that the procedure should be reserved for those patients with end-stage cardiac disease, not suffering from other ailments that would hinder the success of the transplant and for whom the prognosis for survival without transplant is less than one year. Within these broad guidelines, there is some variation among programs in the application of medical criteria as contraindications for surgery. Some transplant programs are accepting patients with ailments that were previously considered adverse to a successful heart transplant (GAO, 1989). These criteria, however, have been examined quite closely and refined as empirical evidence has accumulated and technology and procedures have improved (Hastillo & Hess, 1989).

Most heart transplant programs also consider psychosocial criteria in evaluating patients for transplant surgery (Caplan, 1987; McAleer, Copeland, Fuller, & Copeland, 1985; Olbrisch & Levenson, 1991). Factors such as poor medical compliance, serious alcohol or drug abuse, family dysfunction, psychosis or mental retardation have been proposed by some authors as possible exclusion criteria (Cooper, Lanza, & Barnard, 1984; Freeman, Watts & Karp, 1984; Freeman, Folks & Sokol, 1988; Frierson & Lippman, 1987; House & Thompson, 1988; Kuhn, Myers, Brennan, & Davis et al., 1988; Mai, McKenzie & Kostuk, 1986). Such screening is commonly justified on the argument that severe psychosocial problems contribute to transplant morbidity, if not mortality, because of non-compliance. There is some research suggesting that patients with severe psychosocial problems often have difficulty complying with follow-up appointments, medications, and rehabilitation efforts. (Christopherson & Lunde, 1976; Cooper et al., 1984; Freeman et al., 1988; Kuhn et al., 1988; Mai et al., 1986). There is, however, little empirical evidence that such non-compliant patients are at higher risk for poor medical outcome.

Given the lack of adequate evidence for the predictive validity of psychosocial factors for medical outcomes, it is not surprising that screening practices vary. A survey of 204 active heart transplant centers worldwide (Olbrisch et al., 1991) found wide variations in criteria used and rates of patients refused on psychosocial grounds. The majority of programs required some form of pre-transplant psychosocial evaluation. Most agreed that active schizophrenia, current suicidal intent, history of multiple suicide attempts, dementia, and severe mental retardation were grounds for exclusion. Much less agreement was found on the importance of other psychosocial factors such as cigarette smoking, obesity, noncompliance with medical regimens, recent alcohol or drug abuse, personality disorder, and mild mental retardation. Some authors find the criteria informal, hard to define, primarily subjective and, at times, controversial (Herrick, Mealey, Tischner, & Holland, 1987). Further, the Olbrisch et al. survey also found large variability in the number of patients rejected for transplantation on psychosocial grounds: The proportion ranged from 0% to 37%.

Issues of medical outcome aside, some studies have focused on the psychosocial aspects of the experience of cardiac transplantation itself (Freeman et al., 1988; Frierson et al., 1987; Kuhn et al., 1988; McAleer et al., 1985; Watts, Freeman, & McGriffen, 1984). Much of this literature deals with the impact of the procedure on the patient's emotional and cognitive status, on the recipient's family, and on the process of psychologically adjusting to the transplant. One study (Maricle, Hosenpud, Norman, & Pantelt et al., 1991) examined the possible linkage between pre-transplantation psychological distress and medical outcome in a follow-up study of fifty-eight heart recipients. No such association was found.

The practice of psychosocial screening in selecting candidates for heart transplantation is thus in some flux. Most programs conduct such screening, but there is considerable variation in which factors are considered, how they are weighted, and the formality and consistency of the process. There is relatively little evidence as to the predictive value of psychosocial information available at the time of evaluation for post-transplant mortality or morbidity, for patient's psychological and cognitive adjustment to transplant, or for patient management and compliance issues. In short, there is rather broad agreement that psychosocial criteria are potentially interesting and important, but rather little consensus on exactly how they might be best used.

In the second part of this paper, we report briefly on a study, currently in process, of psychosocial screening procedures in one successful heart transplantation program, that at the Arizona University Medical Center, Tucson, Arizona.

CANDIDATE SELECTION
IN ONE TRANSPLANT PROGRAM

The UMC transplant team consists of approximately twelve members, including cardiac surgeons, cardiologists, internists, transplant coordinators, a social worker, and psychologist. Auxiliary and support staff who may have contact with patients also attend these meetings. The meetings are held weekly, and follow a standard agenda each week. First, current in-patients are discussed. Second, patients who have been seen that week for yearly follow-up evaluations are reviewed. Finally, new candidates are reviewed.

For more than a year the authors have attended these weekly meetings as observers. We have also interviewed all the core team members, exploring a range of both medical and non-medical issues related to the transplant process. A particular focus of these interviews was on identifying psychosocial factors used in screening, and trying to understand how they are used in the process. Finally, we prepared a booklet of fifty "paper patients," summary profiles of imaginary patients varying systematically on seven psychosocial factors identified in the interviews as potentially important. Team members rated each of these "paper patients" on a ten-point scale of overall psychosocial suitability from "Poor" to "Excellent." The process description that follows draws on these observations, interviews, and statistical analysis of the patient profiles.

A comprehensive evaluation is completed on all potential transplant candidates, either on an inpatient or outpatient basis, although the team prefers having patients in-house. The process can be both physically and emotionally taxing as the patient is subjected to a number of diagnostic procedures, examinations, and interviews by various members of the transplant team. This three to four day intensive work-up allows the team to "get to know" the patient in order to select the most appropriate candidates for cardiac transplantation.

All potential candidates are presented and evaluated at the weekly meetings. Because not all patients with cardiac disease are candidates for heart transplantation, the team limits the procedure to those seriously ill patients who stand a reasonable chance of long-term survival with the procedure. Both medical and non-medical factors are discussed.

The medical data are generally presented by either the transplant coordinator in charge of evaluation or by a cardiologist. The medical profile enables the team to determine if the patient is either "too sick" or "not sick enough" for transplantation. The procedure is reserved for those patients with Class III-IV end-stage heart disease for whom the prognosis of survival is less than 12 months.

Medical contraindications have been empirically derived, looking retrospectively at the natural history of cardiac recipients in an attempt to relate outcome after transplantation to risk factors identified in the pre-transplant selection process. Although criteria are now relatively standardized, given the current state of the art of post-transplantation management, these contraindications are subject to change (Copeland, 1990).

A psychosocial evaluation of potential heart transplant recipients is also a part of the preoperative assessment. This evaluation consists of a formalized psychological assessment, including psychosocial interviews, a series of psychological tests, and mental status examination providing both clinical and demographic data. The psychosocial information is presented by the team social worker and psychologist.

This psychosocial assessment helps in the development of individualized patient management plans. It also alerts the team to possible difficulties such as problems adhering to treatment recommendations, traits which may threaten a prolonged working relationship with the team, or psychiatric disorders that might be exacerbated by hospital and surgical stresses. Attempts are made to exclude candidates with a history of behavior patterns or psychiatric illnesses considered likely to interfere significantly with compliance with the demanding post-transplant medical regimen.

Patients with troubling psychosocial factors that are not clearly exclusionary are often assessed for a longer time period. Patients are followed and evaluated through clinic visits, diagnostic medical procedures, and assessment of their comprehension of and compliance with their medical regimens.

Both interviews and observations indicate that most team members give primary attention to medical factors, though all were attentive to some degree to psychosocial factors. Our statistical analyses of the evaluations of the fifty "paper patient" profiles allows us some further insight into this balance. Preliminary analysis of these data supports a number of tentative conclusions:

a. Most members of the team agree that psychosocial factors are important in evaluating a candidate for transplantation. Though importance weights varied across respondents, on average respondents gave psychosocial factors about half as much importance as medical factors in evaluating suitability.

b. As with the importance weights, overall assessments of patient suitability showed reasonable consensus across respondents, though there was important variation between individuals, especially on some specific cases.

c. The seven factors we included in the patient profiles were generally agreed on as important. Though, again, weights differed substantially from one respondent to another, a rough consensus rating would give primary weight to four factors: compliance history, motivation, alcohol/drug use and intelligence; and rather less weight to the other three: social support, smoking and personality.

Our overall impression, drawing on observations, interviews and questionnaire responses, is that there is broad agreement that psychosocial factors are potentially of some importance in screening transplant candidates, but that there is much less agreement on precisely which factors should be considered, what weight should be given to them, and exactly what role they should play in the decision process. These impressions, from a single program, seem broadly consistent with our earlier review of the literature. Psychosocial criteria are attracting considerable interest, but standardized measurement and combination rules, prognostic indices or projected survival curves are some way off.

NEXT STEPS

No settled view of the role of psychosocial factors in transplant screening has yet emerged. Indeed, there is no clear consensus that a standardized procedure is desirable. Authors such as Beresford, Turcotte, Merion, Burtch et al. (1990) can be read as arguing against such standardized procedures, at least in their simplest forms, and in favor of more individualized, case-by-case, flexible assessments.

Our own view is that a degree of standardization is both desirable and achievable. On the former point we claim no special expertise, beyond the obvious arguments about procedural justice and equitable treatment of different patients (see Caplan, 1987; Evans, 1987; Robertson, 1989 for discussion of these issues). Equity may not require that decisions be made in a purely mechanical, formulaic way, but it does appear to call for each case to be considered as comprehensively as the next. Such comprehensive assessment would, in our view, require that similar factors be assessed for all patients, and that any available empirical evidence (such as the weighting of these factor scores that best predicts outcome measures such as survival and quality of life) be also considered. The consideration may well be personalistic and idiosyncratic, but the evidence base, in our view, could be usefully standardized.

With this in mind, we are pursuing two related lines of inquiry. One is to further refine our findings from the patient profiles, with a view to developing a consensus weighting formula for the whole transplant team. This formula, in finished form, could be thought of as preserving the shared judgmental expertise of the team, and thus as a labor-saving device that allows the best and most careful weighing and balancing of factors to be brought to bear uniformly on every case. Our initial data indicate that there is substantial agreement within the team, but that some cases, and some judges, fall outside this consensus. We are working to surface and resolve these disagreements, moving to a consensus judgment model for the whole team.

This consensus model simply externalizes and refines the beliefs of the team members. A second line of our work aims to test these beliefs against empirical data from the outcomes of the cases they evaluate. The UMC Program has now transplanted in excess of 200 patients; they maintain extensive records on each of them. We are working with these files to assess a number of measures of patient outcomes from these files: Survival time, morbidity, quality of life, adequacy of patient self-care, and others. Our aim is to examine the extent to which these outcome measures can be predicted by measures, including psychosocial measures, available at the time of initial evaluation. As with the consensus judgment model, the findings from this empirical prediction model imply no binding constraints on the team's screening decisions. Both models should, however, add to the information available to the team at the decision point.

Our report, then, is of research in progress. Psychosocial evaluation of candidates for heart transplant is an area of clear interest but, as yet, of little consensus. Practices vary widely across (and perhaps within) programs, and there is little hard evidence of the impact of different procedures for patient outcomes. We have described in some detail the procedures we have seen at one successful transplant program, and sketched the tentative findings and likely new directions for our own research with that program. We hope these notes will stimulate further debate and investigation that will move the area to a better understanding of the issues, and an improved use of this knowledge in selecting patients for transplantation.

REFERENCES

Beresford, T. P., Turcotte, J. G., Merion, R., Burtch, G., Blow, F. C., Campbell, D., Brower, K. J., Coffman, K., & Lucey, M. (1990). A rational approach to liver transplantation for the alcoholic patient. *Psychosomatics, 31*(3), 241-253.

Caplan, A. (1987). Equity in the selection of recipients for cardiac transplants. *Circulation. 75*(1), 10-19.

Cate, F. H., & Laudicina, S. S. (1991). Transplantation white paper: Current statistical information about transplantation in America. United Network for Organ Sharing.

Christopherson, L. K. & Lunde, D. T. "Selection of Cardiac Transplant Recipients and their Subsequent Psychosocial Adjustment," in *Seminars in Psychiatry,* 3:1, 36-41, February 1971.

Cooper, D. K., Lanza, R. P., & Barnard, C. N. (1984). Noncompliance in heart transplant recipients. *Heart Transplantation. 3,* 248-253.

Copeland, J. G., Emery, R. W., Levenson, M., M., Icenogle, T. B., Carrier, M., Ott, R. A., Copeland, J. A., McAleer, M. J., & Nicholson, S. M. (1987). Selection of patients for cardiac transplantation. *Circulation. 75*(1), 2-9.

Copeland, J. G. (1990). Selection of patients for cardiac transplantation. *Medical Times, 118*(2), 11-14.

Dec, G. W., Semigran, G. J., & Vlahakes, G. J. (1991). Cardiac transplantation: Current indications and limitations. *Transplantation Proceedings, 23*(4), 2095-2106.

Evans, R. W. & Yagi, J. (1987). Social and medical considerations affecting selection of transplant recipients: The case of heart transplantation, in Cowan, D., Kantorowitz, J., Maskowitz, J., and Rheinstein, P. (Eds.), *Human Organ Transplantation: Societal, Medical-Legal, Regulatory, and Reimbursement Issues,* (pp. 27-41). Ann Arbor: Health Administration Press.

Evans, R. W., Mannien, D. L., Overcast, T. D., Garrison, L. P., Yagi, P., Merrikin, K., & Jonsen, A. R. (1984). *The National Heart Transplantation Study: Final Report,* Volumes 1-5, Battelle Human Affairs Research Centers, Seattle.

Freeman, A. M., Watts, D., & Karp, R. (1984). Evaluation of cardiac transplant candidates: Preliminary observations. *Psychosomatics, 25*(3), 197-207.

Freeman, A. M., Folks, D. G., & Sokol, R. S. (1988). Cardiac transplantation: Clinical correlates of psychiatric outcomes. *Psychosomatics, 29*(1), 47-54.

Freidman, B., Ozminkowski, R. J., & Taylor, J. (1992). Excess demand and patient selection for heart and liver transplantation. *Health Economics Worldwide,* 161-186.

Frierson, R. L. & Lippmann, S.B. (1987). Heart transplant candidates rejected on psychiatric indications. *Psychosomatics, 28*(7), 347-353.

Futterman, L. G. (1988). Cardiac transplantation: A comprehensive nursing perspective. Part 1. *Heart and Lung, 17*(5), 499-632.

General Accounting Office. (1989). Report to the Chairman, Subcommittee on Health, Committee on Ways and Means, House of Representatives. Heart Transplants: Concerns About Cost, Access, and Availability of Donor Organs. GAO/HRD-89-61, Office, Washington, D.C., 2-45.

Hastillo, A., & Hess, M. L. (1989). Who is a suitable candidate for heart transplantation? *Journal of Critical Illness, 4*, 34-44.

Herrick, C. M., Mealey, P. C., Tischner, L. L., & Holland, C.S. (1987). Combined heart failure transplant program: Advantages in assessing medical compliance. *The Journal of Heart Transplantation, 6*, 141-146.

House, R. M., & Thompson, T. L., (1988). Psychiatric aspects of organ transplantation. *Journal of the American Medical Association, 260*(4), 535-539.

Kuhn, W. F., Myers, B., Brennan, F., Davis, M. H., Lippmann, S. B., Gray, L. A., & Pool, G. E. (1988). Psychopathology in heart transplant candidates. *The Journal of Heart Transplantation, 7*(3), 223-226.

Mai, F. M., McKenzie, F. N., & Kostuk, W. J. (1986). Psychiatric aspects of heart transplantation: Preoperative evaluation and postoperative sequelae. *British Medical Journal, 292*, 311-313.

Maricle, R. A., Hosenpud, J. D., Norman, D. J., Pantely, G. A., Cobanoglu, A. M., & Starr, A. (1991). The lack of predictive value of preoperative psychologic distress for postoperative medical outcomes in heart transplant recipients. *The Journal of Heart and Lung Transplantation, 10*(6), 942-947.

McAleer, M. J., Copeland, J., Fuller, J., & Copeland, J. G. (1985). Psychological aspects of heart transplantation. *Heart Transplantation, 4*(2), 232-233.

Robertson, J.A. (1989). Patient Selection for Organ Transplantation: Age, Incarceration, Family Support, and Other Social Factors. *Transplantation Proceedings, 21*(3), 3397-3402.

Olbrisch M. E. & Levenson, J. L. (1991). Psychosocial evaluation of heart transplant candidates: An international survey of process, criteria, and outcomes. *The Journal of Heart and Lung Transplantation, 10*(6), 948-955.

Watts, D., Freeman, A. M., McGriffen, D. G., Kirklin, J. K., McVay, R., & Karp, R. B. (1984). Psychiatric aspects of cardiac transplantation. *Heart Transplantation, 3*, 243-247.

The Ventricular Assist Device Patient

Marilyn R. Cleavinger, MS
Richard G. Smith, MA

SUMMARY. This article provides an overview of ventricular assist devices, which are mechanical pumps that circulate blood within the body. At the present time, these devices are used to provide a "bridge to transplantation" of the heart or to maintain adequate circulation while the heart recovers from injury. Permanent implantation of these devices may soon become a reality. Use of this technology can tremendously impact the recipient's life and adaptation to their circumstances may be difficult. Topics related to the process of adjustment are presented. These include quality of life issues such as optimization of patient care, dealing with the occurrence of complications, limitations in mobility, and possible termination of support. Facing these issues requires great courage and will likely affect personal growth and deepen relationships. Caregivers can be instrumental in helping to meet the basic physical, emotional and spiritual needs of these patients.

INTRODUCTION

Deaths related to cardiovascular disease approach 1,000,000 per year in America.[1] Prevention efforts, surgical procedures and medi-

---

Marilyn R. Cleavinger, MS, is associated with the Artificial Heart Program, University Medical Center, Tucson, AZ 85724.

[Haworth co-indexing entry note]: "The Ventricular Assist Device Patient." Cleavinger, Marilyn R., and Richard G. Smith. Co-published simultaneously in *Journal of Health Care Chaplaincy* (The Haworth Press, Inc.) Vol. 5, No. 1/2, 1993, pp. 45-61; and: *Organ Transplantation in Religious, Ethical and Social Context: No Room for Death* (ed. William R. DeLong) The Haworth Press, Inc., 1993, pp. 45-61. Multiple copies of this article/chapter may be purchased from The Haworth Document Delivery Center. Call 1-800-3-HAWORTH (1-800-342-9678) between 9:00-5:00 (EST) and ask for DOCUMENT DELIVERY CENTER.

© 1993 by The Haworth Press, Inc. All rights reserved.

cal therapy are the routine methods for treating cardiac disease. The availability of transplantation and mechanical circulatory assist devices have expanded the options for treating heart disease. Transplantation was first performed in 1967 as a treatment for end-stage heart disease, however, today the number of potential recipients far exceeds the number of available donor organs. Mechanical devices which can perform the work of the heart hold promise as another alternative for expanding the treatment of heart failure. Estimates indicate that between 17,000 and 35,000 people per year could benefit from ventricular assist device (VAD) use.[2]

VADs are mechanical pumps that help circulate blood within the body. When the native heart no longer provides adequate blood flow to keep the lungs, kidneys, liver, brain or other vital organs working adequately, a VAD may be indicated. VADs are currently used in two major applications. Bridge to transplantation, which provides circulatory support prior to a heart transplant, is one typical use. The other major use of these devices is to provide temporary circulatory support while awaiting recovery following a heart attack, surgery or other type of acute, reversible cardiac injury.

The VADs in use today require external power sources and are intended for temporary use only. VADs suitable for more permanent use are in development now and may soon become a reality. The long-term use of VADs as an alternative to transplantation will further expand the available treatment of chronic heart failure.

HISTORICAL BACKGROUND

Great effort has been expended to develop pumps capable of supporting the failing heart. Several laboratories began work on mechanical circulatory support systems during the 1950s.[2] In 1964, Congress created the Artificial Heart Program and began providing funds for circulatory support device research. The first human implantation of artificial ventricles took place in 1969 at Texas Heart Institute. A total artificial heart (TAH) was implanted as a bridge to transplantation by Dr. Denton A. Cooley when his patient could not be weaned from the heart-lung machine following cardiac surgery. A 47 year old man was maintained for three days on the artificial heart before a donor heart became available.[3] He survived for 36 hours posttransplant before dying of pneumonia.

Significant clinical experience with VADs began in the 1980s. Barney Clark became the first patient to receive a permanent total artificial heart in December of 1982. He survived for 112 days. Early use of the permanent TAH was confined to patients where death was imminent and who were ineligible for cardiac transplant.

Also in 1982, the Thoratec (Berkeley, CA) VAD was successfully used to support a patient in cardiogenic shock. In 1985, a bridge to transplant followed use of a TAH for nine days in a 25 year old man. He survived for nearly five years following his transplant.

DESCRIPTION OF VAD TYPES

VADs can be classified in several ways. VADs pump blood from a single side of the heart when placed as a right or left ventricular assist device (RVAD or LVAD). Biventricular assist devices (BiVADs) attach two pumps to the heart, one to each side. The majority of VADs are designed to leave the native heart in place and carry the blood to and from the pump using special tubes known as cannulae. One type of biventricular assist device, known as the total artificial heart (TAH), is sewn to the upper portion of the heart (atria) after the natural ventricles have been removed.

Pumping can occur at the same rate as the natural heart (synchronous) or at a different rate (asynchronous). The circulatory support provided by the VAD can be total or partial. Pulsatile VADs alternate between filling and ejecting blood and non-pulsatile devices produce continuous blood flow.

Representative types of the VADs currently in clinical use are depicted in Figures 1-6 and described below. Centrifugal pumps and the intra-aortic balloon pump (IABP) are widely available and can be purchased without restriction at the present time. IABP is the most extensively used type of cardiac assist device because of its availability at most community hospitals providing cardiac care.

Other types of VADs are currently available only through Investigational Device Exemptions (IDE). Use of these devices is restricted to centers specifically approved by the VAD manufacturer and the U.S. Food and Drug Administration to study the VAD. The purpose of IDE studies is to determine whether the benefits to the patient and society in general outweigh the risks of using the VAD. The approval process is lengthy and therefore very expensive. Several IDE studies began more than ten years ago, but not until this year did the first IDE VAD become approved for use.

Centrifugal Pumps

Centrifugal pumps (Figure 1) have been in use for many years as the "heart" portion of heart-lung machines used in open-heart surgery. The pump attaches to a console which rapidly spins the inner portion of the pump. As blood enters and flows over the spinning portion of the pump head, it gathers speed and begins to spin also. The resulting swirling motion generates enough pressure to circulate blood through the pump. Blood flow in centrifugal VADs is controlled by the number of revolutions per minute of the inner pump. Centrifugal VADs are relatively inexpensive ($150 per pumphead) and can be used for partial support on the right or left sides of the heart. They require intensive monitoring and that the patient be kept immobilized.

Intra-Aortic Balloon Pump

The intra-aortic balloon pump was the first cardiac assist device to receive widespread use. It was developed during the 1960s and first used clinically in 1968.[4] IABP can increase cardiac output by about 10%.

IABP is most commonly used to assist the left ventricle as shown in Figure 2. A long, slender balloon is placed in the aorta from an artery in the groin. Gas is cycled through the balloon so that it deflates as blood ejects from the left ventricle and inflates while the left ventricle is refilling. This timing pattern reduces the work done by the ventricle, increases the blood pressure and increases blood flow to the heart muscle. Like the centrifugal pump, they are relatively inexpensive ($750 per balloon) and require that the patient be immobilized.

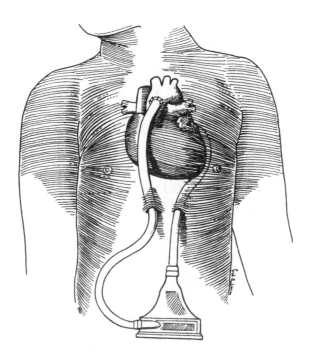

Figure 1. Placement of centrifugal left ventricular
assist device. The pump head attaches to a
drive console.

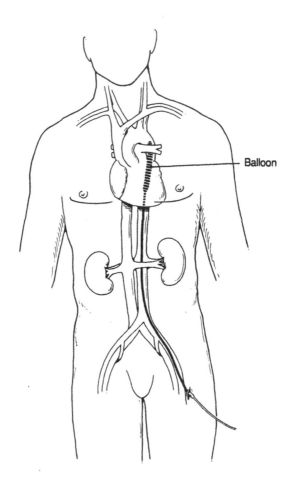

Balloon

Figure 2. Intra-aortic balloon pump placement in the descending aorta. The balloon inflates and deflates during each heartbeat, helping to increase the blood pressure and flow.

Pulsatile Pneumatic VADs

Pneumatic VADS use pressurized air to pump blood. These VADs contain two compartments physically separated by a diaphragm or other flexible barrier. One compartment contains blood; the other air. The wall separating the two compartments moves back and forth, changing the relative size of each compartment, as pressurized air enters and leaves the VAD. Mechanical valves direct the blood chamber to fill as air is exhausted from the VAD. After the VAD fills with blood, the air chamber is pressurized which pushes the diaphragm against the blood chamber to squeeze the blood out of the VAD as shown in Figure 3. The pumping process is regulated by a machine called the controller which is attached to the VADs by drivelines. The patient must remain tethered to the controller until the VAD is removed.

The CardioWest (Tucson, Arizona) total artificial heart, formerly known as the Jarvik or Symbion TAH, shown in Figure 4 is a type of biventricular pneumatic VAD. Its placement within the chest requires removal of the natural ventricles so it is used only for permanent support or bridge to transplantation.

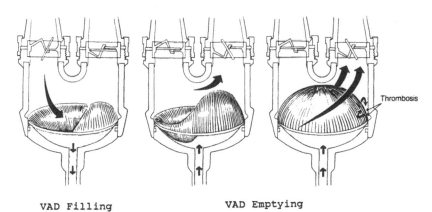

VAD Filling   VAD Emptying

Figure 3. Movement of the diaphragm in a pneumatic VAD during one pump cycle. The diaphragm moves downward to fill and upward to eject blood from the VAD. The two tilting disk artificial valves are shown at the top of the VAD.

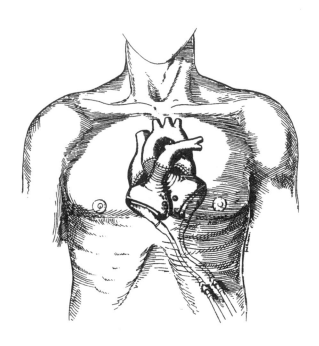

Figure 4. Placement of an artificial heart. The lines which carry the air needed to power the heart come through the skin just below the ribs.

Figure 5 depicts a biventricular pneumatic VAD. These ventricles remain outside the body and are connected to the heart by tubes which are attached to the heart through holes in the abdomen. Despite all the hardware associated with these devices, patients can be mobile and even participate in exercise rehabilitation programs. Single pneumatic VADs can be used on the right or left ventricle which provides this type of VAD a great deal of flexibility. These VADs are expensive, averaging about $12,000 per ventricle. Pneumatic VADs can be used as bridge to transplant or for reversible cardiac injury.

Pulsatile Electromechanical VADs

Electromechanical devices operate in a similar manner to pneumatic devices but do not require air as the power source. The blood compartment is adjacent to moveable plates. These flat plates move toward each other to compress and eject blood from the ventricle and in the opposite direction to fill the pump.

Electromechanical VADs are typically placed within the abdomen (Figure 6). A small driveline exits the abdomen for connection to the controller. Biventricular insertion is not possible due to technical limitations and they are used as left ventricular assist devices only. Cost of these VADs is approximately $25,000.

SURVIVAL RESULTS

Reports published by the voluntary International Registry of the American Society for Artificial Internal Organs and the International Society for Heart Transplantation (ASAIO-ISHT) indicate that as of December 1990, VAD use has been reported in 1,441 people.[5] Implants are categorized as either failure to wean from the heart-lung machine or bridge to transplantation. Total artificial heart use is found only in the bridge to transplantation group but both groups contain all other types of VADs.

Failure to wean from the bypass machine occurs in one to two percent of open-heart surgeries. It can be assumed that none of these patients would have survived postoperatively without the use of a VAD. The ASAIO-ISHT registry results show that 25% of the 965 patients with VADs placed following heart surgery were able to be

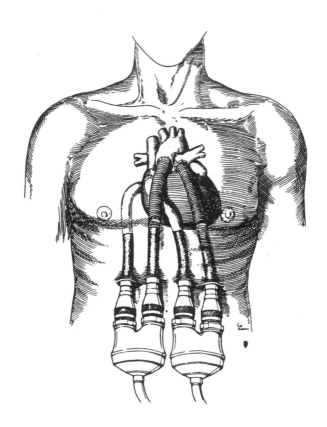

Figure 5. Biventricular pneumatic assist devices. The four tubes (two for each pump) coming through the skin just below the ribs carry blood from the top part of the heart (atria) to the pumps and back into the circulation.

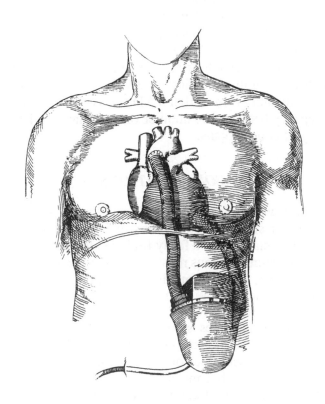

Figure 6. Placement of an electromechanical left
        ventricular assist device. The pump is
        placed below the skin in the abdominal area.

discharged from the hospital after removal of the VAD. The average period of VAD support for failure to wean patients is four days.

Results for the 476 bridge to transplantation patients reported indicate that 45% were discharged from the hospital following cardiac transplantation. The overall survival rate was highest for people receiving only an LVAD (62%) and lowest (35%) for those receiving total artificial hearts. The current average duration of support prior to transplantation is 30 days. This period has increased significantly from earlier VAD use as a result of the increasing discrepancy between the number of potential recipients and the availability of donor organs.

COMPLICATIONS

VADs are used only when cardiac failure is so extreme that expectations for survival without this intervention are very small. VAD use is associated with a fairly high incidence of complications and death. The complications most commonly associated with VAD usage are bleeding, thromboembolism, infection, and failure of other organs such as the kidney or lungs. There have been very few problems with the reliability of the devices.

Once a patient becomes stable on the VAD, the incidence of complications is proportional to the amount of time he remains on VAD support. The occurrence of complications which may delay or preclude VAD removal become a very negative focal point for VAD recipients. One of the most common descriptions from patients and their family members is that of being on a huge emotional roller coaster when complications occur.[6,7]

Some characteristics of VADs are not typically classified as complications but may contribute a great deal to the stress of patients that receive them. Obtaining adequate rest may be complicated by many things: device noise, physical discomfort, anxiety, or interruptions to check device performance or draw blood samples. Placement of VAD tubing or drivelines may limit the patient in finding a comfortable position.

Many VADs produce noise. Moving parts such as mechanical valves, springs or the exhaust from gases used to provide power are typical noise sources. Continual noise from the device can interfere with relaxation and makes some people self-conscious. Alarms designed to enhance the safety of the VAD may sound when the patient strains, such as when using the toilet or even when talking excitedly. This can increase anxiety or feelings of annoyance.

Loss of appetite is a common complaint. Drugs taken to prevent the formation of blood clots or infections may depress appetite. Placement of the VAD in the abdomen or perhaps its continual vibration may produce a constant feeling of fullness. Obtaining adequate nutrition while using a VAD is frequently quite a battle.

PSYCHOSOCIAL ISSUES

People frequently do not have adequate time to think through the implications of VAD implantation before it takes place. It is not a decision one is told to go home and think over. Frequently the decision is made rapidly when some critical event occurs. Many times the patient's condition has deteriorated to the point where death is imminent when the option is presented. He may be mentally confused or not feel he has the time or strength to discuss the matter under these circumstances. The VAD may be placed without the patients knowledge if the decision was made by family members while he was anesthetized during surgery.

Even when there is an opportunity to discuss the situation prior to implantation, the realities of living with a VAD in place can be overwhelming. There may be the presence of strong emotions with conflicting and opposing feelings. Adapting to the circumstances is an ongoing process. Rarely do those involved move directly through typical responses such as shock, anger, and withdrawal to acceptance without cycling back through them in an ebb and flow process.[8]

The first response to the VAD may be very positive, even euphoric. It may seem a miraculous cure has been found just in time to save one from certain death. The patient may recover from the implant surgery and look and feel better than he has in a long time.

If the native heart function recovers and the VAD can be removed, the implant duration may be short and the process relatively straightforward. When recovery occurs, the implant period is usually four to nine days in duration. Bridge to transplantation produces a greater amount of stress and uncertainty. The waiting period prior to transplant is a complete unknown and as patients begin to feel better, they begin to feel more concerned about the sense that they have lost control in their lives.

Attachment to the equipment which patients must remain tethered to is physically and mentally confining. For most VADs the patient must always be accompanied by others anywhere outside his hospital room. Privacy is often hard to come by with frequent interruptions to check the patient's condition and equipment.

There is usually reluctance to discuss the stress of the situation in an attempt to avoid being labelled as a complainer. Patients feel vulnerable and fear that unless they behave well, they may not be cared for or receive a heart transplant. There is anxiety over being a great burden to one's family during the illness, both financially and emotionally. Family members may be reluctant to discuss important issues in an attempt to shield each other from additional worry or to avoid giving the impression that they have lost hope. Tremendous feelings of isolation arise which produce the desire to be left alone along with the fear of being left alone. Well-intentioned caregivers may discourage open communication by trying to always remain upbeat and enthusiastic. An optimistic view of VAD support or technical information about their workings may not be welcomed by the patient. Messages of false hope increase stress and isolation by preventing those involved from expressing their feelings. An atmosphere of security and confidence should be developed, which requires direct and honest medical information and the emotional commitment of the medical staff.[8] The patient should be given control whenever possible and be able to honestly discuss the frustrations from the uncertainty and limitations to this period of his life. Caregivers may need to spend a disproportionate amount of time with these patients and families.

While no two patients are alike and individuality should be recognized, there seem to be some common elements in these patients. Patients frequently express that continuity of care with staff that they feel comfortable with is extremely helpful in reducing their anxiety. Frequent outings to provide exercise or just a change of scenery are usually beneficial (Figure 7). Moving from an intensive

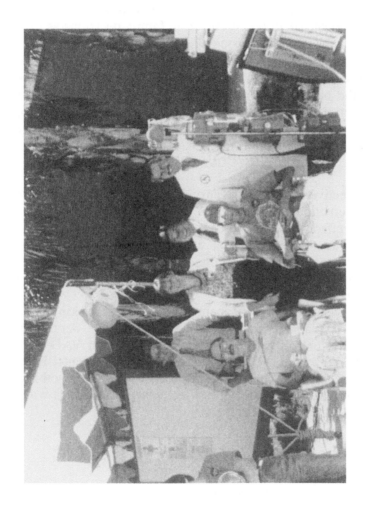

Figure 7. Patient on the total artificial heart (in wheelchair at right) spending time outside on the hospital patio.

59

care environment to quieter quarters where they can attempt to sleep through the night and have more privacy becomes important as the implant duration is extended. The ability to maintain a time schedule and occasionally refuse procedures, food or visitors is important. Patients should be involved in family decisions as much as is practicable. Providing food and encouragement to eat frequently becomes a focus for caregivers. This provides an outlet for those who feel the need to "do something" but may have limited benefit to the patient. Patients and family members may need to share their anxieties separately and should be assisted in doing so.

CONCLUSIONS

A retrospective study of 12 survivors of VAD support asked whether the emotional effects of the assist device were worse than the physical effects. Sixteen percent agreed with the comment and 50% were unsure.[9] However, 83% would recommend a heart assist device to someone who needed one and 67% would reconsent to using the device again if they needed it. The remainder were unsure of their response.

Slow but steady progress is being made toward making VADs more widely available as a treatment for heart disease. As caregivers, we need to understand the dynamics involved in VAD use in order to maximize the support available to these patients. But as Norman Cousins wrote in *Anatomy of an Illness* " . . . nothing a hospital could provide in the way of technological marvels was as helpful as an atmosphere of compassion."[10]

REFERENCES

1. Jaron, D.; Moore, T. W.; & Kresh, J. Y.: Cardiac Assist and Replacement Devices. In Ghista, D. N. (Ed.). *Clinical Cardiac Assessment, Interventions, & Assist Technology.* Adv Cardiovasc Phys. Basel, Karger, Vol. 7 (pp 89-117) 1990.

2. The Working Group on Mechanical Circulatory Support of the National Heart, Lung, & Blood Institute (May 1985). Artificial Heart & Assist Devices: Directions, Needs, Costs, Societal & Ethical Issues. In U. S. Department of Health & Human Services, Public Health Service, National Institutes of Health, *NIH Publication No. 85-2723.*

3. Cooley, D. A.; Hallman, G. L.; Bloodwell, R. D.; Leachman, R. D.; & Milam, J.: First Human Implantation of Cardiac Prosthesis for Staged Total Replacement of the Heart. *Trans. Am. Soc. Artif. Internal Organs 15*:252 (1969).

4. Kantrowitz, A.; Tjonneland, S.; Freed, P. S.; Butner, A. N.; & Sherman, J. L.: Initial Clinical Experience with Intra-aortic Balloon Pumping in Cardiogenic Shock. *J. Am. Med. Assoc. 203*:113-118 (1968a).

5. Shiono, M.; Noon, G. P.; Coleman, C. L.; & Nose, Y.: Overview of Ventricular Assist Devices. In Quaal, S. J. (Ed.). *Cardiac Mechanical Assistance Beyond Balloon Pumping.* Mosby-Year Book, Inc., St. Louis, (pp 25-35) 1992.

6. Farrer, U. L. C.: Total Artificial Heart Experience From the Family's Perspective. In Quaal, S. J. (Ed.). *Cardiac Mechanical Assistance Beyond Balloon Pumping.* Mosby, St. Louis, (pp 329-341) 1992.

7. The Schroeder Family with Martha Barnette, *The Bill Schroeder Story.* William Morrow and Co., Inc., New York (p 234) 1987.

8. Thorstenson, T. A.: Spiritual Support for Patients Requiring Ventricular Assist Devices. In Quaal, S. J. (Ed.). *Cardiac Mechanical Assistance Beyond Balloon Pumping.* Mosby, St. Louis, (pp 342-352) 1992.

9. Ruzevich, S. A.; Swartz, M. T.; Reedy, J.E.; et al. Retrospective Analysis of the Psychologic Effects of Mechanical Circulatory Support. *The Journal of Heart Transplantation,* 9:209-12, 1990.

10. Cousins, N. *Anatomy of an Illness as Perceived by the Patient.* W. W. Norton & Company, Inc., New York, (p 154) 1979.

Waiting:
Pastoral Care to the Cardiac Bridge to Transplant Patient

William R. DeLong, MDiv

Medical technology effects our lives in profound ways. Nowhere is this more clear than in the world of organ transplantation. The modern medical fix of organ transplantation is well publicized in both the popular and academic press. Organ transplantation is not new to us.

Yet, the effects of mechanical devices in the medical arena is not widely known, particularly to those who enter the complex and sophisticated world of modern medicine in search of a cure, of life, in the face of end stage organ disease. Because of the inexperience of those who seek a cure, the importance of the pastoral care giver within this arena is paramount. The hospital chaplain is often the only one on the medical team who is equipped to help patients and families work with and through the drama of organ transplantation.

This article will consider the needs of one group of people within the cardiac transplant population . . . the needs of the patient on

---

William R. DeLong is Chaplain at the University of Arizona Health Sciences Center, Department of Pastoral Care, 1501 N. Campbell Avenue, Tucson, AZ.

[Haworth co-indexing entry note]: "Waiting: Pastoral Care to the Cardiac Bridge to Transplant Patient." DeLong, William R. Co-published simultaneously in *Journal of Health Care Chaplaincy* (The Haworth Press, Inc.) Vol. 5, No. 1/2, 1993, pp. 63-71; and: *Organ Transplantation in Religious, Ethical and Social Context: No Room for Death* (ed. William R. DeLong) The Haworth Press, Inc., 1993, pp. 63-71. Multiple copies of this article/chapter may be purchased from The Haworth Document Delivery Center. Call 1-800-3-HAWORTH (1-800-342-9678) between 9:00-5:00 (EST) and ask for DOCUMENT DELIVERY CENTER.

© 1993 by The Haworth Press, Inc. All rights reserved.

cardiac assist devices. These patients, and their families, are waiting for a donated heart in order for the patient to live. Different from their peers waiting for a heart at home or in a nearby hotel, these patients do not have enough heart function for them to survive even moments without the assistance of a device to pump their blood. So, they are placed in an intensive care unit, attached to a machine which provides enough cardiac profusion, and told to wait. They are in effect, "tied to a machine" (DeLong, 1990).

In this article, I will explore the pastoral issues which are presented with this group of patients. I will trace the course of the patient waiting for cardiac transplantation on a device, suggest that the role of the hospital chaplain is vital to these patients, and finally, provide some methods for the effective pastoral care of these patients.

This technology, known as a bridge to transplant (BTT), is considered medically viable, with an increasing number of centers using the BTT method (Schiedermayer, Shapiro, 1989 and Ruzevich et al., 1990). Unlike other intensive care patients, these BTT patients generally are not ventilated and are alert and oriented. The typical BTT patient is healthy (except for the end stage cardiac disease) has no contra-indications for transplantation, has been financially approved by the institution, is medically stable, and is waiting for the right match with a donor heart. He or she may or may not be with family members for the wait. They are usually motivated for the transplant and have a good knowledge of the transplant process and medical regimes.

The move to place the patient on a "device" may come from two types of thinking. First, the patient may be experiencing an acute cardiac episode where death is emanate. In the mind of the surgeons and the mechanical device engineer, the patient will not survive without this device. The second scenario, is a patient who is slowly going "down-hill" and the cardiac transplant team decides that the intervention with a "device" should be done now while the patient is somewhat healthy instead of waiting until the patient decompensates to a point where nothing more could be done. In either case, the decision to place a patient on a cardiac assist device is a serious intervention with grave consequences for the patient and the family. The need for pastoral care can be profound.

Several types of cardiac assist devices exist. They include the intraaortic balloon pump (IABP), the extracorporeal membrane oxygenation (ECMO), the total artificial heart (TAH), and the ventricular assist devices (VADs), (Ruzevich et al., 1990). My reflections will center on the total artificial heart, and the ventricular assist devices. Both of these mechanical devices have been used in the BTT procedure at this center.

The type of device is important to know because it has an effect on the emotional response of the patient. Devices which leave the patient confined to the bed (such as the IABP) have a more profound impact on the patient than does the VAD. This seems odd since medically, the latter device is considered more serious and invasive. Yet, the increased confinement to the bed has a greater emotional effect on the patient than the knowledge that he may need a more serious device such as a VAD. The hospital chaplain needs to be informed about the various devices in order to understand the kinds of issues which effect the BTT patient.

Psychological adjustment to cardiac transplantation has been divided into six stages (Allender J, Shisslak C, Kaszniak A et al., 1983). They are: the evaluation period, the waiting period, the immediate post-surgical period, the first rejection episode, the recovery period and the hospital discharge. These stages remain for the BTT patient. However, there are several differences in the process in which the BTT patient undergoes. The BTT patient not only undergoes these same stages, but he or she also repeats the stages. So, unlike the "routine" cardiac transplant patient, the BTT patient undergoes the evaluation period twice. Once for admission into the transplant program, and again as the device is being considered. The BTT patient also goes through the immediate post-surgical period twice. Instead of a linear progression through the stages, the BTT patient circles back again and again onto various stages of the "normal" process. Further, the BTT patient is confronted with the "need" for the device. In almost every case, this is viewed by the patient and family as a "setback" and a period of depression is generally seen during the initial phase of adjustment. The stages of psychological or emotional adjustment to transplantation for the BTT patient would look more like this:

1. Initial evaluation period
2. Waiting period
3. precipitating event for the device
4. BTT evaluation period
5. Surgical placement of the device
6. post-surgical period (device)
7. Waiting period with device (BTT) (usually seen as different from the other time)
8. immediate post-surgical period (transplantation)
9. first rejection episode
10. the recovery period
11. the hospital discharge

It will be useful to consider some of these stages from a pastoral perspective in order to understand the emotional process of the BTT patient.

IMPLANTING THE ARTIFICIAL DEVICE

For most BTT patients, the decision to place the device is met with a mixture of emotions. First, the patients are very aware that their health is in jeopardy and that they are "going down hill." For this reason, there is great fear that they will never get their opportunity to receive a transplant, "I won't make it to transplant will I?" This fear can be met with a good deal of hope on the part of families, and transplant staff. Although it is not advocated to present "false hope," it is appropriate and helpful to help these patients understand that the future is uncertain. And, although there is a possibility they will not live to transplantation, there is a chance that they will.

Balancing this need to hope in the face of mounting adversity is very difficult for everyone in the transplant drama. The chaplain plays a very important role here, delineating differences between wishful thinking and other superstitious activity, and genuine hope and realistic faith (DeLong, 1990).

The second predominate emotion at this point is the feeling of relief. Patients who have been struggling with poor health now begin to feel better. The increased cardiac output helps them and for the first time in a long time they feel better. They begin to rely on the device and know that at least it is much more stable than their own heart. Further, they feel that, "now if my real heart goes, at least there is some sort of backup to keep me alive."

It may be difficult for patients to understand and integrate this feeling of relief. Family members who view the implant as a set-back, may have difficulty understanding why the patient is sudden-ly "more himself" and cheerful. These feelings should be brought up with the entire family and a setting to talk it over created to help the family understand why the patient is more relaxed.

Finally, the patient feels committed. The patient, the medical staff have made a commitment to go "all the way" for the patient. When a surgical procedure to implant a device is undertaken, the commit-ment to care for that patient is made clear in a demonstrative way. Patients again feel a sense of relief when they see this kind of commitment. This feeling is pronounced when the total artificial heart (TAH) is selected by the surgeons. The total artificial heart requires that the patient's natural heart be completely removed and implanted with the TAH. In these cases the fear of the patient may be profound, believing that something may go wrong with the de-vice or that they will never get a "real" heart. Pastoral care for these patients should be informed by a thorough understanding of the TAH and the possibilities of such events.

WAITING WITH THE DEVICE

This is by far the most difficult period for the patient and his or her family. The cardiac assist device, although providing some physical stability for the patient, also becomes a constant reminder of the need for the transplant. Unlike other transplant patients wait-ing for a heart and leading a somewhat normal existence outside of the hospital, the BTT patient remains in the ICU with only minimal visits outdoors or even around the hallway.

Four aspects seem to be critical for the BTT patient at this time; depression, control, anger, and denial. Although these feelings do not always move in sequence, in our experience at the University of Arizona Health Sciences Center, we have seen BTT patients enter each of these phases during their waiting period on the device, and generally in this order.

Depression can be expected and is often seen in terms of a lack of hope and a general malaise. The patient often needs a good deal of time alone at this point and the chaplain should be aware of the patient's need to discuss death and poor outcomes. In severe cases, consult with psychiatry has been helpful using mood elevators to enhance the outlook of the patient. Note should be taken to consult with psychiatry as soon as possible because of the delayed effect of drug interventions.

As the time the patient is on the device increases, the patient generally feels the need to control events around his day. In particular when he will take a nap, have teaching sessions, physical therapy, visits from family and friends, etc. We attempt to allow the patient to control these factors as much as possible. One way we do this is creating a schedule and posting it on the wall for the patient to consult at will. Control over daily and routine events gives the patient a feeling of autonomy and self-worth, with little adjustment by the medical team. Even with the schedule posted, it is not uncommon for a physical therapist to come at the appointed time, only to be told by the patient that he is not ready and wants the therapist to come back at a later time. Again, we attempt to accommodate the patient as much as is possible in this area, feeling that it provides much to them with little effect on us.

When control no longer provides the patient with a sense of dignity and worth, and as the patient begins to realize that the wait may be long indeed, he or she generally exhibits a good deal of anger. This may be directed to the nursing staff, the transplant coordinators, the doctors, chaplain or others. The chaplain can be a good person to receive this anger since the patient knows that his or her medical care will not be compromised by getting angry with the chaplain.

Chaplains should be aware of the attempts of patients to disguise their anger by using other emotions to describe their feelings such as "frustration," "upset," "tired of this," etc. As in most instances, giving permission is very important to the patient. The patient needs to learn that the feeling of anger is O.K. but that the way he demonstrates that anger may not be. Providing a physical outlet for the patient can be very important at this point (Daldrup, Butler, Engle, and Greenberg, 1988). Most BTT patients are very grateful to understand that it is O.K. for them to be angry at their disease, their spouses, the nursing staff, God, etc.

Confession is also an important piece of this anger period. Chaplains should be aware that some patients are angry because they feel they are being punished for past events. Forgiveness can be very important for the patient after the anger has been focused and expressed.

Anger is sometimes the result of factors beyond everyone's control. In some instances, the BTT patient is angry about the constant noise of the machine running the device (DeLong, 1989). Again, expressing this in a safe way is very important to the patient and a great relief to the staff.

Finally, during this waiting period, the BTT patient may begin to use denial in a new and deeper sense. This sometimes comes in the form of "what will be will be." BTT patients who have been waiting a number of months may begin to use denial by denying that they will ever get a heart. "I will be living like this forever." "Why don't they just let me go home with this thing (the device)?" The chaplain, again, should be aware that this lines up more with denial than with acceptance. Many times, nurses will respond to me saying that the patient has finally accepted that he is on a device. My experience with this is that the patient is using denial to minimize the emotional effect the prolonged exposure to the device is having on him. This may be accompanied by a good deal of humor. My judgement is that the chaplain should first consider the possibility of denial before rushing to the conclusion that the patient has "accepted" the device.

POST SURGICAL TRANSPLANT PHASE

The final stage of the BTT patient I wish to comment on is the post surgical phase, that is when the transplant has been completed.

Unlike the "routine" transplant patient, the BTT patient has generally waited longer, with more emotional ups and downs. Consequently, when the BTT patient is told that a heart has been found and he is being prepped for surgery, complex emotions begin to surface. By far the most salient emotion is joy and relief. The goal has been reached in their mind. They have made it. The difficult journey is over. This is also the main difficulty for these patients. The journey is in many ways just beginning. The patient needs to understand that a difficult journey is also is about to begin. And, for some patients, this new leg of the journey is more difficult than what they just completed. So, in many ways, the BTT patient is "set-up" for disappointment with the transplant procedure. They believe the transplant can't be worse that what they just went through, and in some cases it is.

The chaplain can help prepare the patient prior to the transplant surgery. This functions in much the same way as anticipatory grief. He is prepared for the new leg of the journey and encouraged to meet it with the same kind of resiliency and faith which he gained from the BTT waiting process. This should be matched with the genuine joy the patient and family is feeling at this time.

Prayer is often very effective at this point. The patient and family is feeling overwhelming feelings of thankfulness and debt (DeLong, 1991). The chaplain by this time has bonded in a profound way with the patient and can share in this joy and thankfulness. It is indeed a blessed moment.

CONCLUSION

My attempt in this paper has been to discuss, from a pastoral perspective, a group of patients with unique needs within the transplant population. Although every transplant center does not use cardiac assist devices, the movement is toward increasing use of these devices. Chaplains in transplant centers should be aware of the special needs of these patients and their families.

With the continued shortage of transplantable organs, more and more physicians are looking at mechanical devices to prolong life when end stage organ disease has occurred. The modern health care chaplain should be aware of the needs of these patients and their families to ensure that the process remains a human and humane experience.

REFERENCES

DeLong, William Riche, "Organ Donation and Hospital Chaplains," *Transplantation*, 50 (1), July, 1990. 25-29.

DeLong, William R., "God's Grace as Gift, A Conceptual Category for Cardiac Transplant Patients," *Journal of Health Care Chaplaincy*, 3:1 (1990b): 23-27.

Allender J., Shisslak C, Kaszniak A. et al. "Stages of Psychological Adjustement Associated with Heart Transplantation," *Heart Transplantation*, 2:228-231, 1983.

Schiedermayer, Shapiro and Ruzevich, in Smith S., ed. *Tissue and Organ Transplantation: Implications for Professional Nursing Practice*, C.V. Mosby, 1990.

Daldrup R., Butler E., Engle D., Greenberg R., *Focused Expressive Psychotherapy*, Gilford Press, 1988.

ETHICAL CONSIDERATIONS

Contesting the Boundary
Between Life and Death:
Organ Transplantation and the Identity
of the Christian Community

M. Therese Lysaught, PhD

INTRODUCTION

Organ transplantation is often discussed without reference to what is actually entailed in the practice itself. In a brief but incisive description, Youngner et al., display the disturbing psychosocial

M. Therese Lysaught is Associate for Religion, Culture, and Health Care Ethics at The Park Ridge Center for the Study of Health, Faith, and Ethics, 676 N. St. Clair, Suite 450, Chicago, IL 60611.

[Haworth co-indexing entry note]: "Contesting the Boundary Between Life and Death: Organ Transplantation and the Identity of the Christian Community." Lysaught, M. Therese. Co-published simultaneously in *Journal of Health Care Chaplaincy* (The Haworth Press, Inc.) Vol. 5, No. 1/2, 1993, pp. 73-89; and: *Organ Transplantation in Religious, Ethical and Social Context: No Room for Death* (ed. William R. DeLong) The Haworth Press, Inc., 1993, pp. 73-89. Multiple copies of this article/chapter may be purchased from The Haworth Document Delivery Center. Call 1-800-3-HAWORTH (1-800-342-9678) between 9:00-5:00 (EST) and ask for DOCUMENT DELIVERY CENTER.

© 1993 by The Haworth Press, Inc. All rights reserved.

effects of the practice of organ extraction on hospital staff. Through vivid images and detail that arise only out of experience, they illustrate ways in which organ transplantation breaches internalized norms of body and medicine:

> Underlying the disturbance felt by staff members are concerns that organ donors are not dead, despite a declaration of brain death, and that the organ-recovery process itself is somehow disrespectful and may indeed kill the donor. . . . Although cadaver organ donors are declared dead, they hardly resemble patients who have died from cardiopulmonary arrest. In fact, they remind us in many ways of living patients. They are warm and retain a healthy color, which is no surprise because their hearts continue to pump oxygenated blood throughout their bodies. Digestion, metabolism, and elimination occur. . . . Maintaining organs for transplantation actually necessitates treating dead patients in many respects as if they were alive. . . . When the potential donors are pronounced dead, we do not follow the customary procedures of turning off the machines, removing the various lines and tubes, and sending the patient to the appropriate place in the hospital–the morgue. Instead, monitoring and intervention continue at maximal levels in order to protect and preserve organs. . . . Should the "patient" have a cardiac arrest, even resuscitation is considered essential . . . . [Moreover, organ retrieval can] represent disturbing deviations from the time-honored rituals and procedures of major surgery. . . . After long hours of arduous surgery, instead of discontinuing the anesthesia and waking the patient, the anesthesiologist must turn off the ventilator, thus halting all the remaining life functions. . . . Operating room personnel may be shocked by the mutilating nature of some procedures, such as the removal of skin or long bones.[1]

Underlying this depiction of organ extraction is a commitment to "the concept of organ donation and transplantation."[2] But, whether one's perspective is committed or critical, the sense of repugnance and disturbance articulated in this passage provides an illuminating point of departure for reflecting theologically on the practice of organ transplantation.

My thesis will be this: the practice of organ transplantation relies on certain cultural understandings of body, suffering, and death that conflict with central self-understandings of the Christian community. In acting on bodies, the practice of organ transplantation reproduces these understandings, strengthening the social order which shares them to the potential deficit of the Christian community. Insofar as the suffering and death of a patient serve as the strongest warrants for this practice, it will be sufficient to examine the understandings of suffering and death embodied in the practice of organ transplantation, identifying how they differ from those affirmed within the Christian community.

SOCIAL ORDER, BODY, AND MEDICINE

Organ transplantation, like many controversial techniques pondered by biomedical ethics, depends on a subtle, evanescent line–etched in flesh–that divides the nearly-deceased from the freshly-deceased. Traversing this line, organ transplantation is made real in the bodies of both the deceased and the suffering ill.

However, rather than attending to this groundedness in the body, arguments for organ transplantation often appeal to social benefit. Drawing on utilitarian reasoning, the "problem" is often identified as one of numbers: authors give figures for the number of transplanted organs versus the numbers needed, or they cite the annual numbers of organs "wasted."[3] Proposed solutions advocate educational efforts that would encourage social altruism and thereby increase various forms of "consent"; these are frequently argued on the basis of the social value of the "gift exchange" dynamic.[4]

The disjunction between this discourse on organ transplantation and its enfleshed reality suggests that free-market economics, utilitarian calculus, or Maussian gift exchange theory overlook a fundamental constant in the equation. The juxtaposition of social arguments and incised bodies suggests that we turn to a discipline which understands the two as linked, namely, a sociology of the body. A sociology of the body analyzes and articulates dynamics by which social orders inscribe, via practices and discourses, normative self-understandings onto bodies and thereby reproduce the social order. I would like to suggest that organ transplantation is one such practice, one whereby contemporary western social orders seek to strengthen their hegemony by reproducing particular understandings of body, self, death and suffering. To explicate this claim requires a summary of the major presuppositions of a sociology of the body.

Sociological perspectives are concerned with two interrelated items: order and power–how social order is constituted and how certain agents acquire the power to maintain that order. To create order, a culture must first differentiate "order" from "disorder." In a given culture, this fundamental polarity will be established and undergirded by analogous oppositional distinctions: clean/unclean, good/bad, productive/unproductive, human/animal, day/night, winter/spring. Dichotomies of this sort help to organize social space, time and relationships and to categorize objects and persons. These distinctions take on normative significance: items correlated with order are considered positive and vice versa. By systematizing this multiplicity of distinctions, normative boundaries are created which circumscribe and structure the social order.

From the perspective of a sociology of the body, the human body is fundamental to this process in three ways. First, the body itself serves as one of "the most intimate and certain of boundaries."[5] Further, it helps generate the dichotomies from which social boundaries derive (e.g., inner/outer, living/dead, self/other). And third, a sociology of the body claims that the body becomes "inscribed" by the same social structures it helps produce; as Martha Reineke has stated, "The social structure is 'reproduced in small' on [the body]."[6] In other words, the surfaces/boundaries of the human body are reciprocally constructed by the dichotomies structuring the boundaries of its culture; they become invested with those cultural meanings. In this way, cultural meanings become "objective," "taken for granted."

Social boundaries themselves are ambiguous, fluid, tensive spaces, the place where ordered and disordered meet. Insofar as social boundaries are created, they can equally be uncreated, dissolved, ruptured. Social boundaries are frequently imaged as an interface of various thicknesses and strengths, a membrane that like the surface of a body contains points of exit/entry; like a body, it is at these points that boundaries are most easily breached and the social order threatened.

As the place where ordered and disordered meet, social boundaries will be peopled with those whose bodies incorporate both order and disorder.[7] These bodies are likewise ambiguous, having assimilated social meanings to lesser degrees or in a state of transition from one degree of order to another. They may, as well, have resisted being fully inscribed by the structures of the social order, have been inscribed by the structures of an alternative social order, or have been inscribed in such a way that they reproduce in their bodies the weaknesses, contradictions, and inconsistencies of the culture. From the perspective of society, ambiguous bodies are 'dangerous,' containing within them potential for challenging and disrupting the distinctions that constitute the social order, insofar as they either do not contribute to its reproduction or directly advocate an alternative social order.

Given the contested and fluid nature of social boundaries, cultures are constantly engaged in the task of monitoring, preserving, maintaining—in the jargon, "reproducing"—their boundaries. A sociology of the body claims that the site of this reproduction is the body itself. Cultural practices monitor the surfaces/boundaries of their constituents' bodies, especially at the points of greatest vulnerability—the orifices:

> ... bodily orifices are especially invested with the symbolism of power and danger. Bodily margins are exposed to disease, assault, and aging. In many cultures, matter that issues from bodily orifices—spittle, blood, milk, urine or feces—attests to that vulnerability. Imbued with symbolism, this matter marks the threat of pollution.[8]

Through practices which monitor these boundaries, cultures "inscribe" their understandings onto bodies. In general, these processes are subtle and perceived as benign, as we are socialized to accept them as "normal"; these would include, for example, practices as diverse as modes of dress, etiquette, transportation. In other cases, these processes of inscription are more literal, overt, painful. When national social power is contested, bodies become the site on which this contest takes place; examples of this would be war and torture.[9] Analogously, within established social orders, certain institutions are mandated to physically, literally, explicitly inscribe social meanings on unruly, recalcitrant, disordered bodies; examples of this would be the incarceration of "criminals" as well as social activists; police brutality against members of marginalized populations; the social toleration of rape and other forms of violence against women.

Institutions which have the ability and social sanction to monitor and control bodies are invested with social power, power which increases in proportion to their control over bodies. Because of their potential to challenge a social order and agents of social power, 'ambiguous' bodies will be the most visible objects that a culture will be concerned to monitor and control in its efforts to maintain social order. But whether a body is marginal or not, it is an object of power. Power, as such, is not a negative, but rather:

> . . . a strategy of relations that gives some individuals and groups the ability to act and keep acting for their own advantage. Power is also the ability to bring about a desired situation, and to prevent the actions of any who would oppose or thwart such desires.[10]

The more fundamental a boundary or more central a power that is being contested by a particular body, the more physical, painful, literal will be the mode of inscription that seeks to exert its reality.

In addition to the penal and legal systems, another institution serves as an agent of social regulation by literally monitoring, touching, and inscribing bodies, namely, medicine. Medicine is charged with overseeing the 'ambiguous' bodies of the sick. Stories of the sick reflect the manner in which well-ordered bodies become "ambiguous," recounting ways in which illness increasingly removes them from the center of social structures toward the margins. "Everyday" activities–working, traveling, shopping, recreation–are disrupted; sick persons are moved out of the public sphere into the private sphere; personal relationships are strained or discontinued; social architectures (e.g., bus steps, distances between home/work/store) become obstacles; voice and rationality become muted or discounted. In this dynamic of illness, one could say that the bodies of the sick become "dis-inscribed"–the traditional social orders inscribed on the body begin to lose their meanings; society's hold over the body begins to dissolve.[11]

Medicine regulates the bodies of the sick in primarily two ways. First, the activities of medicine aim primarily to reinforce dissolving inscriptions. At the same time, medicine initiates a set of practices designed to inscribe a new set of meanings on sick bodies, inscriptions that demarcate the body as one that is sick, one off-center, one moving toward the margins. If medicine is successful in reinforcing culturally normative inscriptions, the inscriptions of illness fade; if not, inscriptions of illness are increasingly reinforced by the bodily practices of medicine. As dis-integration increases, sufferers are removed from our midst to the margins of public space, to the home, to the hospital, to the nursing care facility; increasingly, when that is not enough, there is a movement (namely, advocating euthanasia, assisted-suicide, advanced directives) encouraging that these disordered bodies be moved beyond the boundaries of the human community, beyond the boundary of life and death.

This relationship between body, medicine, and social meanings is crystallized in the practice of organ transplantation. The practice of organ transplantation reflects two trends: (1) that the traditionally stable boundary between "living" and "dead" is not as constant or objective as once thought; and (2) a new set of meanings surrounding this boundary are challenging an established set of meanings. Organ transplantation is one vehicle through which this contest is being waged, in that it literally embodies the new set of meanings. It is premised upon these new meanings and so reflects them; at the same time, it attempts to solidify the objectivity of these meanings by inscribing them on the bodies of both the freshly-deceased and the nearly-deceased.

Most bioethics literature assumes that this traditionally solid boundary (that is, between "living" and "dead") has been destabilized by the advent of new technologies. Technological developments appear to have created a new class of ambiguous bodies, bodies that are "legally" dead but, via technological support, demonstrate physiological function and thereby appear to be "alive," functioning in this manner for a potentially indefinite period of time. But the conspicuous relationship between the redefinition of death (to "brain-death") and organ transplantation indicate that technology is only a symptom of a shift in a deeper set of assumptions which undergirded the traditional boundary, namely, a shift in the relationships between: (1) mind/body and (2) human/transcendent.

First, the practice of organ transplantation requires and reproduces a particular understanding of the relationship between mind and body, namely, a disjunctive dualism. With Descartes and Bacon in the seventeenth century, western cultures marked a shift in their understanding of bodies–bodies came to be seen as machines. This corresponded to a parallel shift in the understanding of nature. No longer understood as teleologically revelatory of and ordered to the service of its creator God, nature came to be regarded as brute, inert, morally neutral matter available to be dissected, manipulated and ultimately mastered, ordered by human purposes to serve human ends. The body, categorized in terms of the natural, became an object for human intervention, manipulation, ownership and transformation.

Alternatively, the mind became the locus of the "person," defined as autonomous and rational. "Persons" understood in this manner became the normative category, that identified with social meaning and ethical significance. Via this distinction, the individual became contingently and not materially related to a body. As such, the definitive activity of a rational being cannot be an action of a body; the definitive activity, rather, becomes that of choosing, expressed by means of voice or consent.

Secondly, correlative to this reorientation in the relationship between mind and body is a shift in the relationship between humanity and the transcendent. As "persons" became ends in themselves, God was displaced; the "person," or more properly the cosmic community of persons, the kingdom of ends, became the transcendent. The *telos* of human life was no longer eternal life, unity with God, the beatific vision, the kingdom of heaven; whether individual or collective, the only *telos* of modern western culture is an end defined relative to "persons," namely, one that is simply *chosen* and in no way constrained, either by God, culture, relationship, nature or one's own body. According to a premier spokesperson in bioethics: "We are alone, and left to our own devices."[12]

These shifts in the relationships between mind/body and human/transcendent translated into shifts in understandings of suffering and death. Pain in the body engenders suffering in persons insofar as it threatens their future–foreshadowing the end of their biological existence, compromising their rationality and autonomy, frustrating autonomous choice of preferences and desires, "dehumanizing." Given that pain and suffering are defined relative to the frustration of the individual *telos,* there is no way for it to be integrated into that *telos* or to serve it in any way. When understood fundamentally as the rebellion of nature against the autonomy of culture, the breach of the autonomy of the self by an action of the body, it is only a problem to be solved, a natural process to be rectified; it must be outlawed, dominated, controlled, and if not these, eliminated via any method possible.

Death, likewise becomes mapped by these understandings of mind/body, human/transcendent. Death is no longer a transition from earthly life to eternal life, a meaningful event. Death is now the end of "personal" existence, the end of rationality, control, autonomy. As such, it can be redefined according to "brain-death" criteria; the end of physical existence is no longer required to be "dead." In a social order which denies the transcendent and identifies the individual as the center of meaning, death will be incomprehensible, that to be staved off as long as possible through any means available, that beyond which there is no meaning.

As has been argued elsewhere, contemporary western social structures and orders rely on these understandings of mind/body and human/transcendent.[13] Suffering and death do not serve the individual or its purposes; they represent the end of the individual. Anything that challenges a public order premised on and constituted by autonomous individuality threatens the stability of its moral meanings and its claims to objective truth. As cultural inscriptions dissolve, those who suffer and face their deaths can begin to question the individual's claims to autonomy, self-sufficiency, and ultimacy; disease, debilitation, degeneration and suffering reveal the contingency of autonomous individuals and the corresponding social order. Unless 'persons' can rid their bodies of the *cause* of suffering, those bodies, in not reproducing the normative ideal of the rational autonomous person, threaten the stability of the social order founded upon autonomy, representing a weakness and point of vulnerability in the boundary. These understandings of person-hood, suffering and death are enacted upon the bodies of organ donors and organ recipients. As one author states, "Most would agree that these donors are no longer 'persons'";[14] this is consid-ered ethically sufficient. Suffering and death so greatly threaten the fabric of contemporary Western culture, that the social response to them must be severe and enfleshed. As power to control suffering and dying translate into social power, so the ability to control the bodies of donors and recipients will become "power asserted in the social sphere to effect social order."[15]

CHRISTIAN PRACTICES, BODIES, AND ALTERNATIVE MEANINGS

In the literature, the evaluation of organ transplantation from religious perspectives varies. At times, organ transplantation is spo-ken of in traditionally religious terms: the "miracle" of organ trans-plantation, the "gift of life." However, when religious perspectives oppose or critique the practice of organ transplantation, they are often castigated as mythic or superstitious.[16] Sensitive to this cri-tique, a number of authors have endeavored to articulate the ways in which religious themes and values support organ donation and transplantation.[17]

An alternative approach would consider the sociological inter-face of religious and medical practices. It has been argued else-where,[18] Christian practices are inherently political and essentially serve to reproduce an alternative social order, namely, the Chris-tian community and the kingdom of God. If society, through organ transplantation, surgically inscribes its meanings onto bodies, the Christian community likewise reproduces its alternative meanings on the bodies of its members but through alternative means, that is, liturgically. But contrary to the practice of organ transplantation, which reproduces a social order characterized by disembodied, autonomous individualism, Christian liturgical practices repro-duce a social order with a different character, namely, the Body of Christ.

Although this claim could and should be displayed in detail, I would like to focus on one particular practice as representative of the effects of Christian liturgical practices: the rites of the sick and dying, especially Communion, Anointing, and Viaticum. What is going on in these practices? What meanings are embodied in the acts of the rites? What form of community is reproduced through their enactment?

We begin by repeating the observation that in illness, pain and suffering, the sick find their bodies gradually "dis-inscribed," losing touch with previous self-understandings, rendering them isolated, marginalized, alienated from their bodies, mute and discounted. Likewise, the self-understandings of one as a member of the Body of Christ are "dis-inscribed" as well. The understandings of the self as related to God who loves, sustains, suffers with, gives life, and can be trusted fade, lose their hold–thus Jesus' bitter lament, "My God, my God, why hast thou forsaken me?"

Thus, through the rites of the sick and dying, the Body of Christ liturgically reinscribes the sufferer with the self-understandings of a member of the Christian community. It does so in a number of ways. First, the rites of the sick and dying are fundamentally liturgical, that is, they are actions that embody and intend the Christian community as a whole. As such, they are communal. This communal dimension assures the sick that, overagainst the social and cultural realities of isolation and marginalization that accompany illness, they are not alone. The rites are understood to unite the sick person with "the assembly from which their sickness has separated them."[19] This bond is reinforced in the ritual actions of touch–the laying on of hands and anointing.

As these rites of the Body of Christ are the actions of God in Christ, they embody God's way of ministering to the sick and suffering. Through the rites, the Body of Christ continues Christ's ministerial mission of comforting, attending to and healing the sick and suffering. In praying with the sick person, the community, in response to God, intercedes for the sick person, praying to God for healing. As the community prays and reads Scripture with the sick, it offers them a language by which to objectify their pains and sufferings, a language of lament that permits their cries of despair to God as well as forms their words of remorse, repentance, supplication and praise; the community serves as their voice in a time when voice can be diminished. And as Jesus ministered to and comforted the sick by touching them, rejecting social taboos that marked the bodies of the sick and 'imperfect' as unclean and ostracized, the Christian community likewise reaches out to the bodies of the sick with a touch intended to heal and comfort.

In addition to continuing Jesus' ministry of healing and comfort, the rites also affirm something more profound, namely, that "When the Church cares for the sick, it serves Christ himself in the suffering members of his Mystical Body."[20] It is not that the sick are simply overlooked in their individuality and attended to 'as if' they were the suffering Jesus; rather, the Church affirms that when the sick suffer, they actually participate in the sufferings of Christ:

> The sick in return offer a sign to the community: In the celebration of the sacrament they give witness to their promises at baptism to die and be buried with Christ. They tell the community that in their present suffering they are prepared to fill up in their flesh what is lacking in Christ's sufferings for the salvation of the world. . . . The sick are assured that their suffering is not "useless" but "has meaning and value for their won salvation and the salvation of the world". . . . and the sick are *believed* to be and seen as productive members of the community, contributing to the welfare of all by associating themselves freely with Christ's passion and death. . . . In the sacrament, the faith of the sick person gives us, the health, a sign–an embodiment–of the words of Paul to Timothy: "You can depend on this: If we have died with him, we shall also live with him. If we hold out to the end, we shall also reign with him." (2 Tm 2:11-12)[21]

Thus, not only do the rites embody God's way of ministering to the sick and suffering; they also embody the meaning and manner of God's suffering.

Not only do the rites challenge the sick not to withdraw from the community, but the rites challenge the Christian community not to exclude the sick. Not only because by attending to the sick and restoring them to health the community hopes to restore the wholeness of the Body of Christ, but rather through these rites, the community is reminded that the Body of Christ is in an important way *constituted* by the sick. The Christian community, recognizing its contingency and utter dependence on God, cannot be closed to the sufferers; it must be open to them, welcoming them, trusting God not only that in incorporating these dangerous bodies their social order will not disintegrate but that these bodies embody the very possibility of the kingdom of God, namely, the sufferings of Christ.

Finally, the rites might be understood as rites of vocation; in these rites, the sick are set apart for a special work, called to a path along which, although not chosen nor foreordained by God, one can follow faithfully. The sick are exhorted not merely to imitate Christ in his sufferings but to actually follow Christ, witnessing God's power, modelling discipleship and so serving as a sign as they "minister to the whole church in their illness."[22]

Thus, through the rites of the sick and dying, the Body of Christ liturgically re-inscribes the sufferer with the self-understandings of a member, reinforcing the unity of the sufferer with Christ in this struggle, as one truly constituted through Christ's Body in relationship with another who can be trusted, namely, God. These liturgical practices embody God's way of ministering to the suffering and sick. Moreover, given the constitutive relationship between the Body of Christ and the bodies of Christians, the sufferings of Christians are given meaning in themselves as they come to be seen as participating in the sufferings of Christ. Through these liturgical practices, Christians are formed in God's way of suffering. Finally, the bodies of the sick and suffering come to be seen not only as an object of the care of the Church but as constitutive for its existence and identity. In sum, through its liturgies the Body of Christ inscribes the bodies of Christians with a *telos* for their living, suffering and dying that differs from the one endorsed by the social order as represented in the practice of organ transplantation, providing them not only with a means to live through suffering and live with those who suffer, but also an end, a meaning, a *telos* for suffering itself which supplies a reason why suffering is not simply to be eliminated but can be lived through.

CONCLUSION

Of course, it is important to say that, contrary to secular stereo-types, Christians are not generally masochists, inviting suffering for its own sake. But these reflections do affirm that for Christians, suffering is not simply to be avoided through any means possible, especially if those means reproduce meanings and orders antitheti-cal to those of the Christian community. The question is whether the practice of organ transplantation is such a means.

Those who counsel and converse with congregants contemplat-ing organ donation and transplantation need to examine the implica-tions of organ transplantation in light of the convictions of the Christian community. They will also need to provide congregants with alternative practices which support and reinforce Christian convictions about the nature of ultimate reality, suffering, and death. The liturgical practices of the Body of Christ perform such practices, practices which are 'counter-productive' to the discourse on suffer-ing in contemporary culture.

Thus, God welcomes into the Body of Christ those who suffer and are sick, comforting them and forming in them the skills to suffer well. It also attends to the bodies of the dead in ways that likewise reproduce the Christian community. The identity of the community that practices these rites understands itself as integrally constituted by those who are sick, suffer, and die, refusing to de-prive them of their status as 'human' or as 'persons' and to relegate them to the margins of the community.

NOTES

1. Youngner et al., 321-322.
2. Ibid., 322.
3. "This year 20,000 people will suffer brain death from trauma. Only 15% of these people will be organ donors. When the rest are buried or cremated, they will take with them approximately 34,000 kidneys, and as many as 17,000 hearts, liv-ers, pancreata, and pairs of lungs. Thus, as many as 100,000 transplantable organs will be lost" (Merz, 3285). See also Prottas and Batten, 121; Youngner et al., 321. Similarly, Manninen and Evans.
4. See Murray (1987) and Murray (1990). See also "Organ Transplantation: Sociocultural Aspects," *Encyclopedia of Bioethics.*
5. Reineke, 247.

6. Ibid.

7. In many cultures, those who attend to or actually touch elements of disor-der–dead bodies, dirt (domestics, garbage collectors, laborers), those who serve the poor–are often closer to the margins than to the center.

8. Reineke, 247.

9. For a fascinating examination of these processes and the way in which they achieve their objectives by enacting their contest on bodies, see Scarry.

10. Finkelstein, 14. She continues: "In these situations the different interests of provider and client are not commonly represented as being in conflict. Indeed, the inherent power and domination of the situation are disguised insofar as the mo-nopoly created by specialist knowledge has been legitimated by sanction of law and professionalism. In the normal transaction between consumer and provider the consumer does not feel exploited by the provider's monopolization of knowl-edge nor abused as his or her experimental subject, because the desire for the product or service has been publicly cultivated while its cost, in monetary and moral terms, has not been so broadly debated or examined. . . . Steven Lukes has argued that this definition of power is extremely subtle because it can direct indi-viduals toward actions the eventual outcomes of which will not necessarily be to their advantage. Such power is also the most difficult to identify because it con-ceals long-term consequences with immediate satisfactions."

11. Just as in instances of pain and suffering, socially inscribed meanings dis-solve, pain and suffering are employed to achieve precisely this effect: to "dis-in-scribe" bodies of certain social meanings, in order to destroy the meanings and (possibly) to reinscribe those bodies with alternative meanings.

12. Engelhardt, 375.

13. References. These are a few that co-exist with many others; the human/transcendent is not often explicated, although it is analogous and important for this analysis.

14. Youngner et al., 324.

15. Reineke, 247.

16. "Religious values complicate the search for usable organs" (Lyon, 54). "Moreover, blacks have many deep-seated fears resulting from religion, myth, and superstition" (Merz, 3286). Prottas and Batten note that those opposed to or-gan donation more often cite religious reasons than those in favor of organ dona-tion or those uncommitted (128).

17. See May (1985), DeLong (1990a) and DeLong (1990b).

18. See Crossan, Hauerwas, Yoder, and Lysaught for interpretations of Je-sus' ministry and the Church as political and social alternatives to their con-temporary orders. This socio-political potency is reflected in the U.S. doctrine of separation of church and state.

19. Pastoral Care of the Sick, no. 46. See also nos. 51, 73.

20. Sacred Congregation for Divine Worship, Decree, *Pastoral Care of the Sick.*

21. National Council of Catholic Bishops, 20-21.

22. Ibid., 41.

REFERENCES

Crossan, John Dominic, "The Life of a Mediterranean Jewish Peasant," *The Christian Century* 108 (December 18-25, 1991): 1194-1200.

DeLong, William Riche, "Organ Donation and Hospital Chaplains," *Transplantation* (July 1990a): 25-29.

DeLong, William R., "God's Grace as Gift: A Conceptual Category for Cardiac Transplant Patients," *Journal of Health Care Chaplaincy* 3:1 (1990b): 23-27.

Engelhardt, H. Tristram, *The Foundations of Bioethics* (New York: Oxford University Press, 1986).

Finkelstein, Joanne, "Biomedicine and Technocratic Power," *Hastings Center Report* 20 (July/August 1990): 13-16.

Hauerwas, Stanley M., *A Community of Character: Toward a Constructive Social Ethic* (Notre Dame, IN: University of Notre Dame Press, 1981).

Lyon, Jeff, "Conundra without End," *Second Opinion* 1(1986): 41-64.

Lysaught, M. Therese, *Sharing Christ's Passion: A Critique of the Role of Suffering in the Discourse of Biomedical Ethics from the Perspective of the Theological Practice of Anointing of the Sick* (Ph.D. diss., Duke University, 1992).

Manninen, Diane L., and Roger W. Evans, "Public Attitudes and Behavior Regarding Organ Donation," *Journal of the American Medical Association* 253:21 (June 7, 1985): 3111-3115.

May, William F., "Religious Justifications for Donating Body Parts," *Hastings Center Report* (February 1985): 38-42.

May, William F., "Attitudes toward the Newly Dead," *Hastings Center Studies* (Will find reference): 3-13.

Merz, Beverly, "The Organ Procurement Problem: Many Causes, No Easy Solutions," *Journal of the American Medical Association* 254:23 (December 20, 1985): 3285-3288.

Murray, Thomas M., "Gifts of the Body and the Needs of Strangers," *Hastings Center Report* 17:2(1987): 30-38.

Murray, Thomas M., "The Poisoned Gift: AIDS and Blood," *The Milbank Quarterly* 68, Suppl. 2(1990): 205-225.

National Council of Catholic Bishops, *Study Text 2: Pastoral Care of the Sick and Dying*, revised ed. (Washington, D.C.: Office of Publishing Services, United States Catholic Conference, 1984).

"Organ Transplantation: Sociocultural Aspects," *Encyclopedia of Bioethics* (New York: The Free Press, 1978): 1166-1169.

Pastoral Care of the Sick: Rites of Anointing and Viaticum in *The Rites of the Catholic Church as Revised by Decree of the Second Vatican Council and Published by the Authority of Pope Paul VI. Study Edition.* English translation prepared by The International Commission on English in the Liturgy. (New York: Pueblo Publishing Co., 1983).

Prottas, Jeffrey M. and Helen Levine Batten, "The Willingness to Give: The Public and the Supply of Transplantable Organs," *Journal of Health Politics, Policy, and Law* 16:1 (Spring 1991): 121-133.

Reineke, Martha J., " 'This is My Body': Reflections on Abjection, Anorexia, and

Medieval Women Mystics," *Journal of the American Academy of Religion* 58 (Summer 1990): 245-265.

Scarry, Elaine, *The Body in Pain: The Making and Unmaking of the World* (New York: Oxford University Press, 1985).

Yoder, John Howard, *The Politics of Jesus* (Reference?).

Youngner, Stuart J., M.D., Martha Allen, R.N., M.S.N., Edward T. Bartlett, Ph.D., Helmut F. Cascorbi, M.D., Ph.D., Toni Hau, M.D., Ph.D., David L. Jackson, M.D., Ph.D., Mary B. Mahowald, Ph.D., and Barbara J. Martin, R.N., B.S.N., M.M., "Psychosocial and Ethical Implications of Organ Retrieval," *New England Journal of Medicine* 313 (August 1, 1985): 321-324.

Are There Any Limits to Scarcity?

Arthur L. Caplan, PhD

As success rates for organ and tissue transplant procedures have improved the criteria for eligibility for receiving a transplant have expanded as well. Twenty years ago the overwhelming majority of kidney or heart transplant recipients were young or middle-aged persons (usually men) with a family, a job, who were psychologically and socially stable and, who had no other major illnesses. Today kidney and heart transplants are being performed routinely on patients in their fifties and sixties, on newborns and young infants, on people suffering from diabetes, retardation and mental illness and upon those who have neither a stable family or supportive social environment.

The size of the demand for organs is not simply a function of how many people have heart, liver, or renal failure on a given day in the United States. While the paradigmatic example of scarcity in the transplant field is a dilemma involving transplant surgeons who must decide who will live when only a single heart, liver or lung is available, scarcity is actually a far more flexible, elastic concept than is implied by such a case (Caplan, 1992a).

The number of people waiting at any given time for an organ or

Arthur L. Caplan is Director of the Center for Biomedical Ethics, University of Minnesota.

[Haworth co-indexing entry note]: "Are There Any Limits to Scarcity?" Caplan, Arthur L. Co-published simultaneously in *Journal of Health Care Chaplaincy* (The Haworth Press, Inc.) Vol. 5, No. 1/2, 1993, pp. 91-98; and: *Organ Transplantation in Religious, Ethical and Social Context: No Room for Death* (ed. William R. DeLong) The Haworth Press, Inc., 1993, pp. 91-98. Multiple copies of this article/chapter may be purchased from The Haworth Document Delivery Center. Call 1-800-3-HAWORTH (1-800-342-9678) between 9:00-5:00 (EST) and ask for DOCUMENT DELIVERY CENTER.

© 1993 by The Haworth Press, Inc. All rights reserved.

tissue in the United States is a function of a number of factors. These factors all interact to produce the kind of rationing scenario with which we are all too familiar. In order to understand how the allocation of organs for transplantation works, and why the 'demand' for organs is far more flexible than it might appear to be, imagine a large funnel. The size of the mouth of the funnel determines how many individuals in the United States are seen as eligible for a transplant at any given time. The size of the funnel mouth is a function of many different variables. Most important for the current system of identifying those in need of transplants are such factors as nationality, access to a doctor and degree of organ or tissue injury, disease or congenital anomaly.

Consider the role nationality and citizenship play in determining the level of demand for organs and tissues and, thus, the size of the scarcity of organs and tissues for transplant. If the admonishment to value all human life equally were taken seriously then our society would put all persons who are in medical need of a liver, heart, pancreas, ligament, cornea or bone for a transplant on our national waiting list regardless of their citizenship. In fact, we do nothing of the sort.

United States citizens are listed almost exclusively on transplant waiting lists. The plight of those in underdeveloped nations who lack access to transplant technologies and even of illegal immigrants to this country is almost always left to these individuals to resolve on their own with very sad results. While the scarcity of organs for transplant is serious, it would be even worse if we really took into account the needs of all those in the world who might benefit from a transplant. Significant expansions of the current transplant waiting list could occur if existing restrictions on the ability to pay or age were relaxed (Caplan, 1992a).

WHAT TO DO ABOUT SCARCITY

The shortage of organs and tissues for transplantation has led researchers to pursue a variety of alternatives, some involving changes in public policy, some involving changes in the sources of substitutes for natural organs. All of them require discussion and debate within the religious community since this is where many persons will turn for counsel and support about these strategies.

In recent years organ transplants of kidneys, liver and pancreas have been attempted using living donors. The University of Chicago has embarked on an effort to test the feasibility of transplanting lobes of livers between biologically related individuals. The University of Minnesota has been experimenting for many years with transplants of the kidney, pancreas and bone marrow between related and unrelated persons. A number of cases have been reported of couples deciding to conceive a child at least partially in the hope that they might find a donor of bone marrow for a sibling or a parent (Kearney and Caplan, 1992). The University of Minnesota, Stanford University and the University of Sao Paolo in Brazil have all embarked on efforts to use living donors of vital organs.

All procedures using living donors involve subjecting the donors to life-threatening risks for no personal therapeutic benefit. While it is surely ethically commendable to decide to give a kidney or a lobe of a lung to a family member or even to a stranger tough questions must be asked about the mental capacity required to make such a choice and the environment that must exist in order to say that someone truly consented or chose to make such a gift.

Consideration is being given at the University of Pittsburgh, Loyala University in Chicago, the University of Cincinnati and other hospitals and medical centers to the use of non-heart-beating donors. This means trying to retrieve organs from those who have died without being on life support.

Since only a small percentage of people now die while attached to life-support only a very small percentage of those who die each year in the United States are candidate for organ donation (many more can donate tissues or corneas). But, if it were possible to find techniques that allowed organs to be taken from those who simply die as a result of heart and respiratory failure, who appear DOA at a hospital or emergency room, the number of potential donors could be greatly increased.

One strategy for trying this is to simply remove kidneys within minutes after cardiac-respiratory death has occurred. While there is no doubt that organs would only be taken from those who are dead, many families might still have their doubts and concerns. Moreover, is it ethical to approach a family in the emergency room within minutes of death in order to request permission for organ retrieval?

Another idea is to try and inject a preservative solution into a cadaver shortly after death to preserve organs. This would give more time to approach families about donation. But, should preservatives be used without the permission of the family? Should such experiments only be tried on those who have signed donor cards? Would the public find such actions too macabre to be ethically acceptable?

Anencephalic infants have been proposed as potential donors of hearts and lungs for other infants in need. The Baby Teresa case in Florida is the most recent in a long line of arguments about the moral acceptability of such a practice.

While these infants will all die and while they cannot think, sense or feel, there should be no doubt that it is only those infants born alive who can be considered as organ donors. Should we change the definition of death to include babies born with most of their brains missing? Or should we change the definition of donor to include babies born with anencephaly (Caplan, 1987)? Either change has obvious and important implications for the theological response to severe disability, parental wishes for the redemption of a tragedy and the meaning of life and death.

Another alternative to cadaver organ transplantation is the development of mechanical or artificial organ substitutes. Kidney dialysis is just such a substitute. The widely publicized efforts to create a total artificial heart, first at the University of Utah and then later at Humana Audubon Hospital in Louisville, Kentucky represent another, albeit failed effort to find an alternative to human organ transplantation as do the effort at the University of Minnesota to create an artificial liver.

Efforts have also been made to modify public policy to encourage more Americans to serve as organ and tissue donors. During the past three years more than forty states, the Federal government and various hospital accrediting agencies have enacted regulations mandating that the option of organ and tissue donation be presented whenever a person dies in a hospital setting (Caplan, Siminoff, Arnold and Virnig, 1992). These efforts have brought a small increase in the number of organs and tissues available for transplantation. But the onset of the AIDS epidemic has severely constrained the number of persons who can be considered as donors. Support for these new laws has lagged in the religious community. And, laudable advances in public health measures such as mandatory seatbelt use and tougher laws against drunk driving have reduced the number of sudden deaths among younger people. Even with a more systematic public campaign to encourage organ and tissue donation the number of donors is likely to remain stable and unlikely to drastically increase.

ANIMALS AS A SOURCE OF ORGANS AND TISSUES

The plight of those dying from end-stage diseases for want of donor organs has led a number of research groups to explore the option of using animals as the source of transplantable organs. Perhaps the most memorable effort to utilize animals was the experiment conducted in 1985 by Dr. Leonard Bailey at Loma Linda University Medical Center in California to try and implant the heart of a baboon into a little baby girl who was born with a fatal congenital heart condition–hypoplastic left heart syndrome. This experiment with Baby Fae did not succeed but it did raise a number of difficult ethical and policy issues which remain unanswered to this day.

Many other research teams including researchers at Loma Linda, the University of Pittsburgh, Stanford, Columbia and Minnesota in the United States and other research groups in England, China, Brazil and France have expressed interest in or have continued research on xenografting. Some, such as Columbia and Loma Linda, are continuing to explore the feasibility of primate to human cardiac transplants. Others such as Pittsburgh have focused their attention on the liver and kidney. Still other programs such as those at Stanford and Minnesota are pursuing lines of research that would allow them to utilize animals other than the higher primates as the source of transplantable organs such as pigs.

These programs and others will aggressively explore the 'xenograft' option in the years to come. Advances will be required on many fronts if animals are to become a viable source of transplantable tissues and organs. Transplant teams must overcome both immunological differences between humans and animals and also show that animal organs can function for many years without problems in human bodies. However, the escalating demand for organs and tissues as well as advances in mechanical substitutes for some organs which permit temporary 'bridging' of children and adults in need of transplants make it certain that society will exert enormous pressure on health care to find alternative sources of implantable organs and tissues and that research on animal sources is a likely avenue for future research and experimentation.

ETHICAL ISSUES RAISED BY XENOGRAFTING

There are many ethical and policy issues raised by the prospect of xenografting. These fall into two general categories, issues associated with basic research and issues associated with clinical experimentation (Caplan, 1992b).

Issues Raised by Basic Research

1. Is it ethical to utilize animal models using species such as pigs and primates in order to study the feasibility of xenografting?
2. What sort of guidelines should animal care and use committees (ACUC) follow in reviewing research proposals?
3. What alternative models exist for exploring the basic mechanisms of xenografting?
4. What sort of findings, both immunological and physiological, would justify shifting from animal to human models in xenografting research?
5. What will the ownership and patent rights be in the area of xenografting techniques?

Issues Raised by Clinical Research

1. Who ought the first subjects of xenografting research be–infants, children, adults, the imminently dying, those who are brain dead, etc.?
2. Which category of organ or tissue ought be the subject of initial research efforts?

3. What sorts of subject selection criteria should be used in 'Phase One' research with respect to xenografting?

4. How can the psychological and ethical issues raised by the use of animal organs best be identified and managed?

5. What sorts of standards should be met before a center undertakes a xenograft?

6. What processes should be in place to assure informed consent and adequate monitoring of subject well-being post-transplant?

7. What are the views and positions of various religious groups concerning xenografting and how ought this bear on subject selection?

8. What procedures ought be in place should the experiment turn out poorly?

9. What sorts of confidentiality and privacy protections should be in place to assure the dignity of human subjects?

All of these issues require a response from the religious and theological community. All too often in fields such as transplantation the religious community has found itself reacting to changes in technology. The reality of scarcity and the need for new sources of organs make it evident that medical research intends to aggressively pursue a number of alternative paths to find answers to the challenge of scarcity including the use of animals as sources of organs and tissues. The time is now for the leaders in the American religious community to proactively engage in a dialogue about the ethics and wisdom of these various paths so that when the time comes they are prepared to respond to the questions, doubts and reservations that will inevitably arise from their congregations and from society as a whole.

REFERENCES

1. Caplan, A. *If I Were a Rich Man Could I Buy a Pancreas and Other Essays on Medical Ethics.* Indiana University Press, 1992.

2. Caplan, A. "Is Xenografting Morally Wrong?" *Transplantation Proceedings,* 24(2), 1992,722-7.

3. Caplan, A. "Should Fetuses or Infants Be Used as Organ Donors?" *Bioethics,* 1(2), 1987, 119-140. (Reprinted in J. Back, ed., *Death/Dying: Opposing Viewpoints,* Greenhaven Press, 1988, 93-9).

4. Caplan, A. and Kearney, W. "Parity for Donation." In: R. Bank and A. Bonnicksen, eds., *Emerging Issues in Biomedical Policy*, New York: Columbia University Press, 1992.

5. Caplan, A., Siminoff, L., Arnold, R., and Virnig, B. "Increasing Organ and Tissue Donation: What are the Obstacles, What are our Options?" In: A. Novello, ed., *Surgeon General's Workshop on Organ Donation*, Washington, HRSA, forthcoming 1992.

Hard at Death's Door

Deborah Mathieu, PhD

Those who strive to prolong human life by replacing malfunctioning body parts ceaselessly pursue new sources for these parts: liver lobes from living donors, brain tissue from fetuses, bone marrow from children specifically conceived for the purpose, transplantable organs from specially-raised primates, and so on. Other methods of increasing the supply of body parts are also being considered, such as changing the definition of death, injecting preservatives into newly dead bodies, and creating more types of artificial organs.

While some people may be dazzled by this potential for sustaining human lives, others–and I count myself among them–are daunted by the profound and perplexing ethical issues involved. Every medical "breakthrough" is a cause for consternation. And it is our own fault: We have been unwilling to undertake a truly comprehensive exploration of the moral issues inherent in the use of organ substitution technologies–we have not even asked some of the most relevant questions–so we have failed to reach consensus on fundamental moral issues. Even the briefest review of recent

---

Deborah Mathieu is Associate Professor of Political Science at the University of Arizona.

[Haworth co-indexing entry note]: "Hard at Death's Door." Mathieu, Deborah. Co-published simultaneously in *Journal of Health Care Chaplaincy* (The Haworth Press, Inc.) Vol. 5, No. 1/2, 1993, pp. 99-108; and: *Organ Transplantation in Religious, Ethical and Social Context: No Room for Death* (ed. William R. DeLong) The Haworth Press, Inc., 1993, pp. 99-108. Multiple copies of this article/chapter may be purchased from The Haworth Document Delivery Center. Call 1-800-3-HAWORTH (1-800-342-9678) between 9:00-5:00 (EST) and ask for DOCUMENT DELIVERY CENTER.

© 1993 by The Haworth Press, Inc. All rights reserved.

cases will demonstrate the moral muddles that pervade the world of organ substitution technology.[1]

"SPARE" PARTS

In October 1984, California surgeons implanted the heart of a seven-month-old baboon into a two-week old baby girl who had been born with hypoplastic left heart syndrome.[2] The child, Baby Fae, lived for almost three weeks with the alien heart, until her body finally rejected it. Her life was perhaps longer (and certainly more uncomfortable) than it would have been without the xenograft.

Perhaps her life would have been even longer, though, had her physicians tried one of the other less radical–albeit still experimental–alternatives. One of the experimental options was a surgical technique developed by Dr. William Norwood and his team, which had been performed–with varying degrees of success–on over a dozen infants. The other experimental option was a transplant from a human donor; a transplant of a human heart was likely to fare better than a transplant of a baboon heart. But Baby Fae's physicians did not seek a human heart, in part because human organ donors for children this young and desperate were (and continue to be) very scarce, and in part because the researchers believed in the therapeutic potential of the xenograft.[3]

This was not the first time an organ from a primate had been transplanted into a human; in the 1960s and 1970s, for instance, researchers tried transplanting the organs from chimpanzees, baboons, and Rhesus monkeys into humans. But because these earlier trials had been so unsuccessful, and little progress had been made since then in crossing the species barrier, the transplantation of a baboon heart into Baby Fae startled many people. It especially startled those who believed that vulnerable Baby Fae had been exploited, that her life had been sacrificed to gratify the research interests of her physicians.[4]

The use of primates as sources for organs raises another troubling ethical issue: Who and what should we include within our moral universe? Do no other animals count morally? Can we be certain that the line should be drawn to include homo sapiens on one side and everything else on the other?[5] Consider, for instance, Dr. Thomas Starzyl's account of an early xenograft with a child:

We got from the Air Force a chimpanzee that was 3 or 4 years old, and the chimpanzee was brought to Denver in a cage and was brought over to my house and had tea. It actually was able to have tea. When it was finished it made some human gestures and so forth. It was so human, it was uncanny. I was really uneasy about taking that little chimpanzee's liver. I would never do it again.[6]

Should he have even done it the first time–especially knowing, as he must have known, that it could not work?

Are there no limits?

UNEXPECTED PARTS

In March 1985, Arizona surgeons removed thirty-three year old Thomas Creighton's diseased heart and replaced it, serially, with three others. Two of the hearts given to Mr. Creighton had been taken from human cadavers; the third was an experimental artificial device known as the "Phoenix heart."

When Mr. Creighton was healthy enough to be a good candidate for a heart transplant, a healthy heart could not be found; so he was given an unstable heart, which failed about 24 hours after transplantation. Mr. Creighton was then placed on a heart-lung machine while the medical team searched for another transplantable heart. When none could be located, he was placed on the artificial Phoenix heart. The device was still in its early experimental stages (designed for implantation into a calf, and thus too large to fit inside Mr. Creighton's chest cavity), and had not been approved by the federal government for use in humans.[7]

Mr. Creighton survived for approximately 21 hours without a human heart (10 hours on the heart-lung machine and 11 hours on the Phoenix heart). But his condition deteriorated so badly during this time that he almost certainly would not survive, no matter what was done for him. Nonetheless, he was given a very scarce resource: a healthy human heart transplant. He died about 12 hours later.

The implantation of an artificial heart was not one of the treatment options discussed with Mr. Creighton prior to his operation;

the decision to implant the artificial device was made only after the first donor heart had failed and no other could be found. Therefore, not only had Mr. Creighton not consented to receive an experimental device, he had not even known that it was a possibility. This is troubling.[8] It is a basic tenet of good medical practice that a competent patient must give his or her informed, voluntary consent to all medical procedures; this holds especially true for risky, experimental procedures, such as implantation of an artificial heart. Indeed, an important element of all codes of ethics governing research with human subjects is the requirement that the researcher obtain the voluntary, informed consent of the competent subject before proceeding with the experiment.

But it was not just the use of the Phoenix heart that was problematic; the use of the human hearts also triggers concern. The scarcity of transplantable hearts is sadly illustrated by the woeful condition of the first heart transplanted into Mr. Creighton: the heart had been taken from an accident victim who had been hospitalized for several days with fevers and fluctuating blood pressure and who, one of the transplant surgeons stated, "wasn't what we would call an excellent donor candidate." But it was the best heart that could be found. Yet after he was no longer able to use it, Mr. Creighton was given a perfectly good heart–a scarce resource that no doubt could have benefited someone else more.

These three issues–the value of the informed consent of the patient, the persistent shortage of transplantable organs, and the just allocation of health care goods and services–recur again and again. Consider, for example, twenty-six-year old Susan Fowler, whose autoimmune hepatitis had destroyed her liver. In October 1992, her physicians embarked on an unprecedented effort to keep her alive: unable to find a suitable human liver, they transplanted a pig liver into her instead. Like Thomas Creighton, Ms. Fowler was not aware that she might become the subject of an experiment; she was comatose when the possibility was considered.[9]

And like Thomas Creighton's artificial heart, Ms. Fowler's xenograft was intended to be temporary. Her name was moved to the top of the waiting list for a human liver. She was given priority, apparently, because she was so close to death: the xenograft was unstable, and her severe brain swelling could not be controlled. But although a suitable organ was located within hours, it was used on someone else; Ms. Fowler died before the transplantation could be performed.

But should the physicians even have sought a donor liver? Given the unrelenting shortage of transplantable organs, would it have been fair to others in need to give one of these very scarce resources to a woman whose brain swelling was killing her? And if she should not receive a new liver because of the extremely low chance that she would benefit from it, then could the xenograft–which was intended to keep her alive while a new liver was sought–be justified? Are there no limits?

Surely Ms. Fowler should have been given the opportunity to accept or reject such an extraordinary–and experimental–measure. And surely, given the persistent shortage of transplantable organs, we should take great care to give them only to patients we have good reason to believe will benefit from them.

PAYING FOR PARTS

Sheri Dexter, a 30 year old Arizona resident, learned in June 1990 that she suffered from chronic myelogenous leukemia. Because the anticancer drugs she took to combat the disease also destroyed her bone marrow, Ms. Dexter decided to pursue the possibility of receiving an allogenic bone marrow transplant (a transplant of the bone marrow from a matched donor).[10] The average cost of the procedure, however, was $170,000, and was not covered by Arizona's Medicaid program, of which Ms. Dexter was a beneficiary. Unable to afford the price of the procedure on her own, Ms. Dexter sued the Arizona Health Care Cost Containment System (AHCCCS), asking the court to order the state to pay for the bone marrow transplant.

The district court ruled in Ms. Dexter's favor, on the grounds that AHCCCS had discriminated against her in refusing to pay for an allogenic bone marrow transplant since it would have paid for an autologous bone marrow transplant (a process in which a patient's bone marrow is removed and then returned after chemotherapy). Ms. Dexter underwent the transplant a week later–using closely matched marrow donated by her sister–and AHCCCS paid for it.

Unfortunately, her body and the new marrow were fatally incompatible, and she lived for only about three more months.[11]

Ms. Dexter had a compelling claim when she sued AHCCCS: she was dying, and a treatment existed which might save her life–a treatment she would receive only if AHCCCS would pay for it. But was AHCCCS wrong to deny her?

Like all other Medicaid programs, AHCCCS does not provide all health care goods and services to all needy people. Indeed, like all other Medicaid programs, it rations both benefits and beneficiaries. AHCCCS has been, in fact, outstanding in both respects.[12] As a result, Arizona remains at the bottom of most lists when it comes to providing adequate health care goods and services for its residents.

Ms. Dexter argued that AHCCCS should expand its benefits–specifically, to include the expensive, technologically sophisticated procedure she needed. Perhaps Ms. Dexter was correct, and AHCCCS should continue to deny basic health care to needy people in order to add expensive last-ditch treatments for those already under its wing. Perhaps, then, AHCCCS should also consider paying for other transplant procedures it currently denies: pancreas transplants, for instance, and liver transplants for adults. Or perhaps AHCCCS should move in a different direction: perhaps it should include more children, or make greater efforts to treat more pregnant women and so reduce Arizona's lamentable infant mortality rate, or hasten its plans to treat mentally ill adults. There is only one certainty: AHCCCS will never provide everything for everyone.

The dilemma raised by Sheri Dexter's need for a bone marrow transplant raises, once again, the issue of the allocation of scarce resources, but this time in a wider context. Her case illustrates the fact that we should consider the opportunity costs of embracing each new technology. That is, we need to consider whether supporting this new technology will jeopardize other goods we wish to support: there may be other forms of health care that can produce more benefit for the same expenditure, and there may be some non-health related goods that are equally vital. Health is important, but it is not, after all, the only thing of value.

Thus health care goods and services will always be rationed. We need, then, to choose a principle of allocation. And we need to consider organ substitution technology within the context of this principle. What should it be: "The most for the most?" "Everything for a few?" Or something else?

Are we any closer to settling this issue than we were forty years ago? The vague and ambiguous health care programs espoused by both George Bush and Bill Clinton in the last election could lead one to conclude that we still have far to go. And we will make little progress so long as those involved refuse even to contemplate one of the logical alternatives: abandonment of "extraordinary" last-ditch efforts to prolong a relatively few human lives so that those resources can enhance the lives of many more people.

RECOGNIZING LIMITS

The woeful state of affairs described in the case studies above is a result of several troubling factors. First, we have failed to resolve many of the moral issues that confront us: where we should obtain the replacement body parts and what we may do with them remain highly controversial and problematic. This is disquieting; for if we have not reached consensus on the ethical quandaries that have been vexing us for the many decades in which physicians have been transplanting human organs and tissues, what makes us think that we will have any greater success resolving the batch of ethical problems that awaits us?

But a lack of moral consensus is not the whole explanation, for surely we have come to agree on *some* ethical issues over the years. The problem here is that all too often the resolution of ethical questions exists only in the abstract. We give lip service to the importance of informed consent and fairness and doing no harm and protecting the vulnerable, but ultimately these values are outweighed by two seemingly irresistible goals: postponing death and "advancing" medicine. And so long as these goals remain compelling, the moral niceties–of informed consent and fairness and protecting the vulnerable and so on–will be slighted.

These two goals will continue to prod us on as long as we remain unwilling to challenge the moral value of "life" at any cost in any form. Not only is this blindspot dangerous, but it is especially odd within the context of a health care system that allows so many premature deaths to occur because of lack of access to basic medical care. Do we really need an artificial liver more than we need decent prenatal care?

Real ethical progress depends on our willingness to ask all of the relevant questions. And perhaps the most important–and certainly the most basic–concerns the incredible lengths to which we will go to avoid death. Our quest to prolong human life at almost any cost alarmed Paul Ramsey over two decades ago, and his response was to call for a radical change in our attitude toward death. We should, he argued, adopt a "less triumphalist attitude toward death."[13] Otherwise death is always to be avoided, or at least postponed; and no cost is too great when it comes to forestalling the death of a human; and there are no limits to what is allowed in attempting to prolong a human life. And the number of incidents like the ones described above–which amount to a series of uncontrolled and largely unjustified experiments on unsuspecting patients–will multiply.

Surely we should set principled limits. To do so, though, we must first recognize that life is not the ultimate good and death is not an unqualified evil. And those who know this best–the leaders of the religious community–are our best teachers. With your continued help perhaps one day even the most zealous researchers will come to see that devising ever new methods of forestalling the inevitable–and neglecting in the process certain basic moral rules–will only continue to add, in Baron Lyndhurst's words, "another terror to death."

NOTES

1. The world of organ and tissue substitution technology is not an anomaly within the U.S. health care system; it simply puts a special spin on problems that pervade the whole system.

2. A rare defect in which the left side of the heart is unable to pump enough blood to support life for more than a few weeks.

3. The final option, of course, was to let the child die.

4. See, e.g., Charles Krauthammer, "The Using of Baby Fae," *Time* 24(23): 87-88, 1984; George Annas, "Baby Fae: The 'Anything Goes' School of Human Experimentation," *Hastings Center Report* 15: 15-17, February 1985. For other concerns, see, e.g., Kenneth Vaux, "Baby Fae and Human Wholeness," *Christian Century* 101: 1144-1145, December 1984; John C. Fletcher, John A. Robertson, Michael R. Harrison, "Primates and Anencephalics as Sources for Pediatric Organ Transplants," *Fetal Therapy* 1: 150-164, 1986.

5. For arguments that our views of other animals are tragically mistaken, see: James Rachels, *Created from Animals* (New York: Oxford University Press,

1990); Tom Regan, *The Case for Animal Rights* (Berkeley: University of California Press, 1983); Peter Singer, *Animal Liberation* (New York: Random House, 1975).

6. Testimony before the Subcommittee on Investigations and Oversight of the Committee on Science and Technology, U.S. House of Representatives, 98 Congress, 1st Session, April 1983, p. 123.

Notably, Dr. Starzyl is currently overseeing a transplant program which uses the organs of baboons and a new experimental anti-rejection drug.

7. Officials of the Food and Drug Administration investigated the matter and determined that no sanctions were in order because the Phoenix heart had been used in a "very unique emergency situation." For criticisms of their position, see Leslie Francis, "Legitimate Emergencies, Experimentation, and Scientific Disobedience," in Deborah Mathieu, ed., *Organ Substitution Technology* (Boulder: Westview Press, 1988), 243-256.

8. This concern is mitigated somewhat by the fact that his parents gave their approval for the implantation while their son was incompetent to do so. But it is important to note that Mr. Creighton himself, who was not a minor, should have been the one to decide whether to resort to that extreme and experimental method of sustaining life. One wonders what Mr. Creighton was led to expect from the original heart transplant–whether he had realized that the transplant might not work. And one wonders what steps he had agreed to should something go wrong. One also has to wonder how Mr. Creighton would have reacted had he awakened to find himself permanently attached to the Phoenix heart (a real possibility, given the propensity of patients with artificial hearts to suffer severe brain seizures and infections, which usually preclude transplantation of another heart).

9. Her parents, like those of Thomas Creighton, gave permission in her stead.

10. A search of a pool of 20,000 potential donors may be needed to find a single match; the success rate for an allogenic bone marrow transplant varies with the disease being treated–from 45 percent to better than 70 percent. National Marrow Donor Program, "The Chance of a Lifetime," 1989 pamphlet.

11. Although continuing to pay for more of these expensive procedures, AHCCCS appealed the case. [After Ms. Dexter's death, the Arizona Chapter of the Leukemia Society of America intervened as appellee. The appeal was heard in April 1992 by three judges of the Ninth Circuit Court of Appeals]. This time the court ruled in favor of AHCCCS, declaring that "The [federal] statute applicable to payments for organ transplants . . . does not make payments mandatory." In response, Arizona state legislators amended the AHCCCS statutes to require AHCCCS to pay for some allogenic bone marrow transplants.

12. During AHCCCS's first several years, for instance, the federal government allowed it to refuse to pay for some major health care benefits that all other state Medicaid programs were required to cover: home health services, room-and-board payments for long-term care, family-planning services, nurse midwife services, and services for the chronically mentally ill. Over time, most of

these benefits have been incorporated into the AHCCCS program, although mental health care for adults remains woefully inadequate (e.g., AHCCCS did not begin paying for the treatment of seriously mentally ill adults until November 1992, and still does not pay for the treatment of those who are less seriously ill). And as its eligibility limits demonstrate, AHCCCS was designed for the poorest of Arizona's poor:

Family Size	Monthly Income Limit (AFDC)
2	$233
3	$293
4	$353
5	$412

'AFDC' refers to Aid to Families with Dependent Children, the government program that helps support women with minor children. Beneficiaries of this program are automatically beneficiaries of AHCCCS.

13. Paul Ramsey, *The Patient as Person* (New Haven: Yale University Press, 1970), p. 221.

Organ Donation:
A Catholic and Interfaith Perspective
on Its Ethical Warrants
and Contemporary Public Policy Concerns

Jeremiah McCarthy, PhD

The dramatic case of Theresa Ann Campo Pearson discloses the great promise as well as the wrenching ethical and social dilemmas presented by the technology of organ donation and transplantation. This infant, tragically born without the upper hemispheres of the brain and doomed to die, presented the nation with the plight of grieving parents seeking to recover some semblance of meaning and purpose from her impending death by making her available for organ donation. In large measure, the media focus was a reprise of a similar episode at Loma Linda University Medical Center which resulted in trial protocols to retrieve organs from anencephalics like Theresa (a program which is now suspended).[1] What are the moral justifications for organ donation, and what are the limits that should be observed as society continues to avail itself of this burgeoning technical marvel?

Jeremiah McCarthy is Dean of St. John's seminary in Camarillo, CA.

[Haworth co-indexing entry note]: "Organ Donation: A Catholic and Interfaith Perspective on Its Ethical Warrants and Contemporary Public Policy Concerns." McCarthy, Jeremiah. Co-published simultaneously in *Journal of Health Care Chaplaincy* (The Haworth Press, Inc.) Vol. 5, No. 1/2, 1993, pp. 109-121; and: *Organ Transplantation in Religious, Ethical and Social Context: No Room for Death* (ed. William R. DeLong) The Haworth Press, Inc., 1993, pp. 109-121. Multiple copies of this article/chapter may be purchased from The Haworth Document Delivery Center. Call 1-800- 3-HAWORTH (1-800-342-9678) between 9:00-5:00 (EST) and ask for DOCUMENT DELIVERY CENTER.

© 1993 by The Haworth Press, Inc. All rights reserved.

In this essay, I propose to examine three issues. First of all, I will review the ethical warrants for organ donation from a Catholic perspective with attention to insights from different religious viewpoints including Jewish, Buddhist and Islamic traditions. In the second part of the essay, I shall examine some of the dilemmas surrounding proposals to increase the supply of organs for transplantation. These issues involve questions both of access to the supply of organs as well as the allocation of this scarce resource. Finally, I offer a constructive proposal for health care chaplains who are involved in these discussions with family members suggesting that attention to the religious themes of covenant and the common good are important resources for positive education programs.

AN INTERFAITH PERSPECTIVE ON ORGAN DONATION

Public policy discussions of organ donation are filled with philosophical distinctions concerning informed consent and the ethical criteria governing the formulas for the acquisition and disposition of "human body parts" (HBP's: a helpful term coined by ethicist James Childress to encompass not only solid organs such as hearts, lungs, kidneys and livers, but also tissues such as corneas and bone marrow).[2] The religious justifications for organ donation are equally compelling and a review of some of these considerations is valuable for purposes of public policy conversations. As a Roman Catholic seminary professor who has been involved in interfaith and ecumenical health care settings, I will attempt to reflect my own faith tradition and to represent as fairly as possible (though not exhaustively) Jewish, Islamic and Buddhist perspectives.

Roman Catholic moral thought draws upon an important philosophical underpinning, namely the tradition of natural law reasoning. This tradition, which traces its ancestry to Stoic philosophy through the Roman legal tradition, and the recovery of Aristotle for Western philosophy in the work of Thomas Aquinas in the thirteenth century, may be described as "right reason reflecting on reality."[3] A cardinal commitment of natural law reasoning is its reliance upon the virtue of prudence, a skill which is developed by critical examination of issues and the wisdom of shared experience. Such a process generates a set of common convictions about shared moral values that is continually tested by experience, new data, and continuing discernment.

Rather than a monolithic abstraction, natural law scholars view natural law as a critical process of discernment about the moral enterprise, and a process which forges bridges among competing perspectives. In the area of medical ethics, for example, the Roman Catholic tradition has contributed important distinctions to guide withdrawal of treatment decisions (e.g., the distinction between proportionate and disproportionate medical means), as well as a body of reflection drawn from case studies to guide moral assessment in a wide range of medical issues.

The discussion of organ donation is particularly illustrative of this tradition. Prior to the successful kidney transplant performed by Dr. Joseph Murray at Peter Bent Brigham Hospital in December, 1954, Catholic moralists were debating the ethics of this procedure.[4] As a source of moral guidance, moralists drew upon the principle of totality which governs the proper disposition of the body. In other words, the traditional understanding of the principle of totality was that it protected the integrity, the "wholeness" or "totality" of the body. Given this construction of the principle, it was difficult to extend it to embrace the emerging technology of organ donation since the donor would have to undergo significant impairment of his or her own "totality" in order to benefit another person. Faced with this issue, several moralists lead by Gerald Kelly S.J., suggested another route of moral justification which would complement the principle of totality. Kelly's appeal was to the principle of charity, or other-regarding love, as a means of justifying the donation of an organ.

However, this endorsement of organ donation was also qualified by additional considerations. While the desire to donate was commendable, the donor was not to undergo such a procedure if the donor were to suffer not only anatomical impairment (e.g., the loss of a functioning kidney), but also loss of functional integrity, that is, the capacity to perform crucial physical functions necessary for health and well-being. For example, a donor would not be permitted to donate a functioning cornea while alive since the cornea of a healthy eye is necessary for the function of binocular vision.[5] Moreover, careful consideration must be given to an assessment of the benefits and burdens of a transplant procedure. Accordingly, moralists Ashley and O'Rouke suggest the following principles: serious need on the part of the recipient for which there is no alternative therapy; no functional impairment of the donor; the risk undertaken by the donor is appropriately measured or proportionate to the expected outcome; and the action of the donor complies with the canons of informed and free consent.[6]

In light of the above analysis, it becomes clear why organ donation has enjoyed the approbation of papal teaching. Pope Pius XII is representative of this commitment in the following passage:[7]

> . . . a person may will to dispose of his body and to destine it to ends that are useful, morally irreproachable and even noble. (among them the desire to aid the sick and the suffering)

Biblical warrants for this position can be cited from the Book of Genesis 1:27 which states that human beings are fashioned in the "image and likeness" of the Creator. Correlative to this insight is the observation that the sanctity of human life entails an obligation of stewardship and care for the gift of life. Since all human beings are fashioned in the likeness of the Creator, each person is to be treated with equal regard and with rights or claims that ensue from this fundamental sense of value. According to Pope John XXIII:[8]

> Every human being has the right to life, to bodily integrity, and to the means which are necessary and suitable for the proper development of life.

A crucial theme in Catholic social theory flows from this conviction, namely the solidarity of the human family which is captured in the principle articulated by the American Catholic bishops in their pastoral letter on the U.S. economy, namely the "dignity of the human person in community."[9] As applied to the issue of organ donation, this principle provides support for the life-sustaining relationship that is expressed in the donation of human body parts.

David Thomasma, bioethicist at Loyola University Medical Center, argues further that a proper understanding of Catholic worship strengthens the bonds among persons and supports the obligation to donate organs. As Catholics reverently recall the action of Christ in surrendering his body and blood for the community in the celebration of the Eucharist, Thomasma contends that this dramatic action is a paradigm for reminding the community of the obligation to surrender our own bodies for the benefit of others. Hence, organ donation enjoys not only secular but also religious support from the community of faith.[10]

The most recent papal pronouncement on organ donation is that of Pope John Paul II in an address given to the first international congress of the Society of Organ Sharing, June 20, 1991. In this address, the pope endorsed organ donation as "that sincere gift of self which expresses our constitutive calling to love and communion."[11] The papal address acutely recognizes the shortage in transplantable organs and the current situation in the United States where more than 23,000 individuals are waiting to receive a transplant.[12] Increasing the supply of organs is one of the most widely debated issues in the medical-ethical literature, and will be more fully addressed in part two of this essay.

In a helpful taxonomy of religious objections as well as justifications for organ donation, W. F. May accentuates the positive affirmation of the body that is distinctive of Christian and Jewish traditions.[13] This positive assessment leads both communities to affirm the value of organ donation. Jewish law reflects a distinctive interplay of both Scripture (the Written Law) and the Oral Law (which reflects centuries of rabbinic commentary on the Written Law). According to this tradition, an individual can donate his or her organs to save the life of another because "his blood is no redder than theirs."[14] This dynamic quality of Jewish Law, "halachah" ("the walking") leads D.W. Weiss to observe that transplantation of organs must be undertaken in a context of profound respect for the donor and the recipient of the organs:[15]

> Dominant halachic opinion holds that a reasonable risk may be assumed voluntarily–any form of coercion is interdicted–when it is probable that the transplant will save, or prolong, the life of the recipient; and, that the donor may place himself in even significant hazard when imminent death of the patient seems otherwise certain.

Moreover, the critical process of halachic reasoning provides a source for evaluating the new questions confronting organ donation today. The allocation of resources leads Rabbi Fred Rosner to the view that a policy of "first come, first served," or pure medical criteria might be more preferable in Judaism.[16] D.W. Weiss also suggests that the benefits of organ donation need to be continually re-examined lest a policy of "somatic engineering" compromise the dignity and the infinite value of the human person.[17]

In a joint statement issued by the Roman Catholic-Jewish Respect Life Committee of the Archdiocese of Los Angeles, both communities concurred that the issue of equal access to health care is of paramount importance for every individual, and that the allocation of resources, including organs for transplantation, should be based not on a determination of "quality" of life or social value, but rather on the basis of the "equality" of life.[18]

In a careful review of Islamic religious law, A.A. Sachedina summarizes the emerging consensus of Muslim scholars:[19]

> It is possible to summarize Islamic views on organ transplant by pointing out the underlying principle of saving human life. Whereas the limited right of a person is recognized on his/her body, which is a trust from God and as such is to be preserved and respected, donation of organs from both living and dead has been regarded as permissible in the jurisprudence. However, the prerequisite in the case of a living person is that his/her life is not endangered, whereas in the case of a dead person there must exist his last will of testament permitting thus, or the permission of his relatives.

Sachedina also concludes that there is an array of questions yet to be addressed by Islamic scholars, a situation attributable to the historical and geographic location of the Islamic world, and the developing skills of Islamic physicians in searching the sources for approaches to contemporary ethical issues.[20]

K.T. Tsuji, commenting on the Buddhist view of organ donation, observes that although there is no single tradition on this question, the Buddhist view of the world as one of fundamental interdependence provides an important moral warrant for the practice of organ transplantation. According to Tsuji:[21]

> An enlightened view of the body and its relation to the whole universe will immeasurably enhance the quality of human life. As medical science progresses, organ transplantation will be perfected and more and more people suffering from various ailments will be helped by enlightened donors.

The above review of different religious traditions accentuates a common thread of support for the practice of organ donation, but with reservations concerning particular ethical questions raised by this new technology. In the next section of the paper, I will briefly review the most pressing ethical concerns, and suggest some approaches from a Catholic perspective.

INCREASING THE SUPPLY OF ORGANS FOR TRANSPLANTATION–ISSUES OF PROCUREMENT AND DISTRIBUTION

Many early ethical concerns related to procurement of organs from cadavers have been largely resolved through the application of medical criteria which call for the cessation of all brain activity, including the lower brain stem. The case of Theresa Pearson, however, has raised the issue of the use of anencephalic newborns as candidates for organ donation. Due to the difficulty of diagnosing brain death in these infants, proposals have been made to re-define the criteria for brain death so that these infants with functioning lower-brain stems can serve as organ donors. However, the implications of such a policy revision have met with sharp criticism in the literature. In an extensive critique of this proposal, Alan Shewmon and colleagues argue forcefully that instrumentalizing these infants in order to benefit others deprives them of their inherent dignity and protectability as human subjects. Moreover, the pool of available organs is not likely to increase, nor is there sufficient justification to impose unnecessary medical measures in order to maintain the viability of these infants for transplantation.[22]

I support the analysis of Shewmon and his colleagues and judge that serious harm to the principle of respect for the dignity of the human person would result from a change in current protections for anencephalic newborns. Nonetheless, the critical issue remains, how can we increase the available supply of organs? With more than 20,000 people awaiting a transplant, can we rely on altruism as the motive for organ donation?[23] Should consideration be given to the sale of organs?

Currently, according to the Organ Transplant Act of 1984 passed by the U.S. Congress, sales in human organs are specifically prohibited. John R. Williams reviews the arguments for organ sales and concludes that efforts should be increased to educate the public about the social value of organ donation. The chief objection to human organ sales is the commodification of the body and the implications of a free market economy which would set a price on human life. While both proponents and opponents invoke different moral values, namely equality and individual liberty, Williams contends:[24]

> The opponents of organ sales are dissatisfied with this individ-
> ualistic approach to political economy. They consider the so-
> cial nature of human beings to be equal, if not prior to their
> individuality, and therefore, must always be balanced against
> social responsibilities and the needs of others. Society func-
> tions best on the basis of co-operation rather than competition.
> Social forms of regulation are needed to prevent powerful
> individuals and groups from pursuing their self-interest at the
> expense of the vulnerable . . .This line of reasoning leads to the
> rejection of the sale of organs and the call for legislation to
> prevent it.

Kevin O'Rourke argues that organ sales should be prohibited on the basis that organ donation is not an obligation in strict justice, but should be chosen "in the freedom of charity."[25] An additional argument drawn from the principle of distributive justice, a princi-ple which seeks to maximize the fairness of the claims of all to basic societal goods, argues in a similar vein that the poor and disenfran-chised would be at risk and tempted to sell their organs to the highest bidder. An alternative approach is to seek means to improve the voluntary system of organ donation.

Various suggestions have been made to increase the supply of organs, among them different versions of "presumed consent" and "required request." Presumed consent would empower physicians to remove organs unless specific refusal has been expressed. Required request protocols would broaden efforts to educate the public to participate in organ donation. James Childress argues that required request procedures are in the best interests of public policy since they minimize the danger of coercion and the creation of a negative climate for organ transplantation:[26]

> In general, I argued for laws and policies to maintain and facilitate express donation of organs by individuals and their families. Such laws and policies, including required request, should be given adequate time to determine their effectiveness before moving to other major alternatives, such as presumed donation and sales. Presumed donation is not ethically unacceptable in principle, but for it to be ethically acceptable in practice, vigorous educational efforts would be required in order to ensure that a person's silence reflects a decision to donate rather than a lack of understanding.

I find this line of reasoning to be persuasive and commensurate with the values of fairness and equity. These same values are also at stake in the question of allocation of scarce organs. While criteria are in place concerning tissue matching, waiting lists and sharing of organs in the various regional transplant centers, more delineation of these criteria is necessary. In particular, a more focused public policy debate needs to take place concerning the fiscal commitment to health care in this country. While an appraisal of insurance mechanisms would go beyond the focus of this paper, it is surely preferable that medical criteria rather than arbitrary social worth criteria should prevail in discussions of organ allocation as well as other health care resources.[27]

In summary, a Catholic perspective on the question of increasing the supply of organs for donation emphasizes the importance of distributive justice so that all have fair access to the pool of available organs, and the importance of respect for the dignity of the individual person so that commodification of the body is not furthered by recourse to the sale of organs. Moreover, efforts should be undertaken to maximize the value of altruism so that organ donation does not become subjected to impersonal and potentially inequitable market forces. Finally, some implications for health care chaplains follow from this essay which I address in the concluding section.

THEMES OF COVENANT AND THE COMMON GOOD AS RESOURCES FOR EDUCATION ON ORGAN DONATION

With the advent of required request legislation in many states, chaplains often find themselves in a position to assist family members with a decision about organ donation. Often, the family is grieving the loss of a loved one, and the approach that is taken must be sensitive to the complex emotional dynamics that are operative. I suggest that the religious theme of covenant and its correlative moral analogue, the notion of the common good, can provide important resources for communicating the positive value of organ donation.

The motif of the covenant is pervasive in the Hebrew and Christian Scriptures and is eloquent in its depiction of the Creator as an intimate Lord who cares for human beings and sustains them in moments of grief and loss. Language, therefore, which draws upon this powerful biblical imagery may be more conducive both emotionally and spiritually to the family members who must decide. To make this suggestion, however, is not to endorse a manipulative use of religious language in order to maneuver a family into a decision for organ transplantation.

My point, rather, is to suggest that focusing upon the constructive meaning of the covenant invites a different vision of what organ donation means. Ethics is not simply about "decisions" or "choices," it is also about the overarching "vision" of the moral good to which we aspire as moral agents. Covenant loyalty which accentuates God's loving care for humanity is far more attuned to the reality (and, I would argue, the spiritual meaning of organ donation) than referring to organ donation as "harvesting" which diminishes the human and spiritual significance of the act of donation.

In addition, the covenant reminds us powerfully of the communal bonds which link us to the Creator and to one another. The "common good" is a notion in Catholic social theory which is drawn from this biblical motif in order to highlight the investment of all in the goods which facilitate human flourishing and growth. The expansive interdependence conveyed by this notion can help communicate the largesse that is fostered by an organ donation. In their searching critique of American values, Robert Bellah and his colleagues at the University of California, Berkeley, have identified a spirit of "corrosive individualism" as a problematic concern.[28] Recovering a deepened sense of our shared humanity and solidarity with one another is sorely needed as attested by the recent riots in Los Angeles in May, 1992.

To speak of organ donation in terms suggested by covenant loyalty and the notion of the "common good" may provide a helpful vehicle for public education and increased commitment to alleviate the critical shortage in available organs. Moreover, recourse to such language also provides an important ethical caveat that needs to inform the development of organ transplant technology. As the history of kidney transplantation has indicated, particularly with the development of cyclo-sporine to minimize tissue rejection, organ donation is a cost-effective alternative to long-term dialysis. Nonetheless, the ethical question that confronts all of medicine, not just organ transplantation, is the issue of the "technological imperative." In other words, serious attention must be given to the limits of technology for the benefit of human beings. Resources must be marshalled for the benefit of all, and care needs to be taken so that technology genuinely serves human well-being rather than vice-versa. The covenant theme reminds us of these limits and can keep us anchored as we seek to increase the supply of organs for donation.

In conclusion, I have endeavored to present a Catholic viewpoint, sensitive to the insights of other faith traditions, and have offered some ethical reflection on efforts to increase the supply of organs. Other ethical issues, including the use of fetal tissue from elective abortions have not been addressed (though I am opposed to such a practice on ethical and public policy grounds) in an effort to focus on the religious themes of the covenant and the common good as valuable assets for the educational efforts of health care chaplains in promoting the societal good of organ donation.

NOTES

1. Shewmon, Alan, Capron Alexander et al., "The Use of Anencephalic Infants as Organ Sources, A Critique," *Journal of the American Medical Association*, 261(12), March 23/31, 1989:1773-1782. For more references, please see note 22.

2. James Childress, "Ethical Criteria for Procuring and Distributing Organs for Transplantation," *Journal of Health Politics, Policy and Law,* 14(1), Spring 1989:87-114, at page 87.

3. Jeremiah J. McCarthy and Judith Caron, *Medical Ethics: A Catholic Guide to Health Care Decisions,* (Liguori, Mo.: Liguori Publications, 1990): pages 15-16.

4. Ashley, Benedict and O'Rourke, Kevin, *Health Care Ethics,* (St. Louis: Catholic Health Association, third edition, 1989): pages 304-312. For a detailed ethical history of organ transplantation, see Arnold G. Diethelm, "Ethical Decisions in the History of Organ Transplantation," *Annals of Surgery* 211(5): May, 1990, pp. 505-520, at p. 507.

5. Ashley, Benedict, and O'Rourke, Kevin, *Health Care Ethics: A Theological Analysis,* op. cit., pages 304-307.

6. Ibid., pp. 307-308.

7. Pius XII, "Tissue Transplantation," May 14, 1956, in *Medical Ethics: Sources of Catholic Teachings,* edited by Kevin O'Rourke and Philip Boyle, (St. Louis: Catholic Health Association, c.1989): 214.

8. Pope John XXIII, Pacem in Terris, as cited in "The Allocation of Scarce Medical Resources," Rosner, Sordillo et al., *New York State Journal of Medicine* 90/11 (November, 1990): 556.

9. National Conference of Catholic Bishops, *Economic Justice for All* (Washington, D.C., United States Catholic Conference): 1986.

10. David C. Thomasma, "The Quest for Organ Donors: A Theological Response," *Health Progress,* (September, 1988): 23-24.

11. News Release from the National Kidney Foundation, New York, June 25,1991.

12. Ibid.

13. W.F. May, "Religious Obstacles and Warrants for the Donation of Body Parts," *Transplantation Proceedings* XX no.1, Suppl 1 (February, 1988): 1079-1083.

14. Pesachim 25b, as cited in Rosner, Sordillo et al., "The Allocation of Scarce Medical Resources," op. cit., p.556.

15. D. W. Weiss, "Organ Transplantation, Medical Ethics, and Jewish Law," *Transplantation Proceedings,* XX, No. 1, Suppl 1 (February), 1988:1071-1075, at p. 1074-1075.

16. Rosner, Sardillo, op.cit., p.556.

17. Weiss, op. cit., p. 1075.

18. *A Covenant of Care: A Jewish-Catholic Reflection on the Religious Contribution to Health Care and Medical Ethics,* (Los Angeles: The Roman Catholic-Jewish Respect Life Committee of the Archdiocese of Los Angeles, 1986) p. 17.

19. A.A. Sachedina, "Islamic Views on Organ Transplantation," *Transplantation Proceedings*, XX, No. 1, Suppl 1 (February), 1988: 1084-1088, at p. 1088.

20. Ibid.

21. Ibid.

22. Shewmon et al., op. cit. The position of James Walters Ph.D. of Loma Linda University, who supports the transplantation of organs from anencephalic neonates, is discussed in *The Journal of Pediatrics,* 115 No. 5 Part I, November 1989:825-829. Ferhaan Ahmad M.D., supports the critique of Shewmon and colleagues in his essay, "Anencephalic Infants as organ donors: Beware the slippery slope," *Canadian Medical Association Journal* 146(2) (January 15, 1992): 236-245.

23. Ake Grenvik, "Ethical Dilemmas in organ donation and transplantation," *Critical Care Medicine,* 16 No. 10 (October, 1988):1012-1019. An interesting assessment of this question is also available from Dolores O'Connell RN, "Ethical Implications of organ transplantation," *Critical Care Nursing Quarterly,* 13(4): 1-7, 1991. Kathleen Barzizza RN offers a helpful update on the experience of the United Network for Organ Sharing (UNOS) in her essay, "Ethical Questions in organ transplantation still not answered," *AORN Journal,* 52(5): 1076-1080, November, 1990.

24. John R. Williams, "Human Organ Sales," *Annals, Royal College of Physicians and Surgeons of Canada,* 18(5): 401-405, September, 1985.

25. Kevin O'Rourke, "On Selling Organs," *Ethical Issues in Health Care,* (St. Louis University Medical Center), 4 (December, 1979).

26. James F. Childress, op. cit., p. 111.

27. Helpful discussions of these issues are developed in the following essays: Martin Benjamin, "Medical Ethics and Economics of Organ Transplantation," *Health Progress,* (March, 1988): 47-53; J.B. Dossetor, "Ethical Issues in Organ Allocation," *Transplantation Proceedings*, XX (1), Suppl 1 (February, 1988): 1053-1058; "Organ Transplants: Small Supply vs. Great Demand, Who Gives, Who Receives, and Who Pays?" *Issues,* 1(2): September, 1986: 1-8.

28. Bellah, Robert and Colleagues, *Habits of the Heart: Individualism and Commitment in American Life,* (Berkeley: University of California Press, 1985).

PASTORAL AND THEOLOGICAL PERSPECTIVES

The Discerning Heart: The Psalms as Pastoral Resource in Ministry to Potential Organ Recipients and Their Families

Donald Capps, PhD

Because the word "plant" is a part of the word "transplant," we may assume that the word "transplant" originally had agricultural connotations, and that it referred to the act of removing a plant from one location to another, where it would be more likely to grow and

Donald Capps is William Harte Felmeth Professor of Pastoral Theology at Princeton Theological Seminary, Princeton, NJ.

[Haworth co-indexing entry note]: "The Discerning Heart: The Psalms as Pastoral Resource in Ministry to Potential Organ Recipients and Their Families." Capps, Donald. Co-published simultaneously in *Journal of Health Care Chaplaincy* (The Haworth Press, Inc.) Vol. 5, No. 1/2, 1993, pp. 123-136; and: *Organ Transplantation in Religious, Ethical and Social Context: No Room for Death* (ed. William R. DeLong) The Haworth Press, Inc., 1993, pp. 123-136. Multiple copies of this article/chapter may be purchased from The Haworth Document Delivery Center. Call 1-800-3-HAWORTH (1-800-342-9678) between 9:00-5:00 (EST) and ask for DOCUMENT DELIVERY CENTER.

© 1993 by The Haworth Press, Inc. All rights reserved.

123

flourish, Later, the word "transplant" would be applied–more metaphorically–to humans, usually groups of humans, who would move or be removed from one place and resettle in another. As in the first, so in this second meaning of the word, there is the implication of great risk, as the transplantation could lead not to a renewal of life but to traumatization, despair, and even death. Also implied in both meanings is a sense of cautious hopefulness. The transplantation may succeed: the new soil and the new land may prove to be hospitable, and the plant may grow as never before, and the people may live richer and fuller lives than they could ever have imagined. In a sense, the risk and the hope go hand in hand. Transplantations of plants and peoples carry great risk precisely because they engender hopes which may or may not prove to be well-founded.

A third sense in which the word "transplant" is commonly used is, of course, the medical sense, where it has to do with the transfer of a vital organ or vital tissue from one individual to another, or from one part of the body to another. In this article, I will have mainly in mind the transfer of vital organs from one individual to another individual, though transplantations from one part of the body to another (e.g., bone and skin grafts) are not entirely unrelated to what I will have to say here about pastoral care.

The medical or surgical meaning of "transplant" has much the same sense of risk and hope that attends the other meanings, as there is much the same possibility that the organ will find its new environment an inhospitable one, and the same cautious hopefulness that the transplanted organ will not be rejected. But the surgical meaning of "transplant" differs from the other two in one very important respect. In the other meanings, emphasis is placed primarily on the survival of that which is being transplanted, whether a plant or a people. In the medical or surgical meaning, greater emphasis is placed on the survival of the individual who receives the new organ. An organ is chosen that appears to "fit" the person who is receiving it, but there is always the risk of the body's rejection of the organ. In such cases, it is not the organ that is lamented, but the person whose life the organ was meant to save. It is the "host" whose survival is at stake, and the new organ is being implanted precisely so that the "host" may live and not die.

This way of looking at the transplantation process reframes the more traditional understandings of the term. It is as if a plant were moved from one place to another because the soil in the new location needed the plant for its own enrichment, or as if a people were moved from one region of the earth to another because the new region needed these new immigrants to secure its own survival. Until the medical meaning of the term came into being, the emphasis was on that which was being transplanted, whether a plant or an immigrant people. Now that the medical meaning has become the most prevalent one, emphasis is being placed on the recipient, the one who is the "object" of the transplant, and what benefits this individual is expected to receive from the transplantation. This raises a host of new questions, ethical and strategic, as to the circumstances under which an organ transplant is an appropriate surgical procedure. When heart transplants were first attempted in the 1960s, serious questions were raised not only about whether surgeons were attempting to "play God," but also about the very real possibility that the patient and his family were being exploited by these surgeons in the interests of scientific research, as not only was the patient's life expectancy severely limited but the quality of the life that the transplant afforded was also marginal at best.

However, my reflections here on organ transplants are not concerned with the ethical issues involved. Others will be writing more systematically and more penetratingly about these matters. Instead, I propose to address the transplantation issue from a pastoral theological frame of reference, centering on certain biblical understandings of the heart, and on the pastoral care implications of these biblical insights.

THE HEART: OUR VITALIST ORGAN

The type of surgical transplant that has received the most publicity over the years is the heart transplant. This publicity is due, in part, to the fact that the heart is such a vital organ. If the transplant does not have the desired effect, death will surely follow. Yet, the same can be said of other vital organs, such as the kidney or the liver. There is something special about the heart, owing, in part, to the symbolic meanings we attach to it, especially that it is associated with life itself. As Richard Selzer points out in *Mortal Lessons: Notes on the Art of Surgery* (1974), there was a time in human history when the liver "was regarded as the center of vitality, the source of all mental and emotional activity, nay, the seat of the soul itself" (p. 64). It was considered by the ancients to be the organ through which the gods spoke, a belief that supported divination practices, as priests would slit open the belly of a sheep or goat and read the markings on the animal's liver. However, with

> the separation of medicine from the apron strings of religion and the rise of anatomy as a study in itself, the liver was toppled from its central role and the heart was elevated to the chair of emotions and intellect. The brain is even more recently in the money, and still has not overcome the heart as the seat of the intellect, as witness the quaint reference to learning something "by heart." (p. 65)

The heart, Selzer concludes, has become the "aristocrat" of the vital organs. It is also pure theatre,

> throbbing in its cage palpably as any nightingale. It quickens in response to the emotions. Let danger threaten, and the thrilling heart skips a beat or two and tightrope-walks arrhythmically before lurching back into the forceful thump of fight or flight. And all the while we feel it–hear it even–we, its stage and its audience. (p. 63)

Perhaps if the liver was originally associated with life itself (liver = live), could it be that the heart came to be associated with life itself because it was evident that life had gone out of a person when the heart could no longer be heard (heart = hear)? In any event, the heart came to be associated with inner strength and vitality: "Ancient man slew his enemy, then fell upon the corpse to cut out his heart, which he ate with gusto, for it was well understood that to devour the slain enemy's heart was to take upon oneself the strength, valor and skill of the vanquished" (p. 63). Here, the "host" takes into himself the strength and vitality of the one whose life has come to a premature and violent end. But acquiring the life strength of another by ingesting his heart was not the only way in which another's heart might bring strength to others. Selzer cites the practice of the adoration of the heart of a saint among Christian devotees:

> It was not the livers or brains or entrails of saints that were lifted from the body in sublimest autopsy, it was the heart, thus snipped and cradled into worshipful palms, then soaked in wine and herbs and set into silver reliquaries for the veneration. (p. 63)

Selzer adds: "It follows quite naturally that love should choose such an organ for its bower. In the absence of love, the canker gnaws it; when love blooms therein, the heart dances and *tremor cordis* is upon one" (p. 63). The heart, then, is associated with the emotions, especially the "higher" emotions of courage, devotion, and love. According to Selzer, it was Plato who "placed the higher emotions, such as courage, squarely above the diaphragm, and situated the baser appetites below, especially in the liver, where they squat like furry beasts even today, as is indicated in the term 'lily-livered,' or 'choleric,' or worse, 'bilious'" (pp. 65-66).

THE HEART OF THE PSALMS

For the ancient Hebrews, the heart was, indeed, the center of emotion, but it was far more than this. It was also the seat of wisdom (the locus of discernment), and the region in which intentions—both good and bad—are conceived. It is also the locus of desire. The book of Psalms has over one hundred references to the heart, which may roughly be divided into those that speak of the "desires" of the heart, those that concern the "intentions" of the heart, those that view the heart as a place of discernment, and those that refer to the various "emotions" of the heart. Examples of psalms that view the heart as a place in which desires are held and entertained are 21:2: "Thou hast given him his heart's desire, and hast not withheld the request of his lips"; and 37:4: "Take delight in the Lord, and he will give you the desires of your heart." Illustrative of psalms that view the heart as a place in which intentions are conceived are 66:18: "If I had cherished iniquity in my heart, the

Lord would not have listened"; and 17:3: "If thou triest my heart, if thou visitest me by night, if thou testest me, thou wilt find no wickedness in me." Where the intentions of the heart are concerned, a distinction is made between a pure heart and a duplicitous heart: "Truly God is good to the upright, to those who are pure in heart" (73:2) and "Everyone utters lies to his neighbor; with flattering lips and a double heart they speak" (12:2) or "His speech was smoother than butter, yet war was in his heart" (55:21).

Examples of psalms that view the heart as a seat of discernment are 16:7: "I bless the Lord who gives me counsel; in the night also my heart instructs me"; and "I commune with my heart in the night; I meditate and search my spirit (77:6). Examples of psalms that view the heart as the center of emotions are 4:7: "Thou hast put more joy in my heart than others have when their grain and wine abound"; and 73:21-22: "When my soul was embittered, when I was pricked in heart, I was stupid and ignorant, I was like a beast toward thee."

The psalms also refer to the heart's current condition or status. The heart may be broken: "Insults have broken my heart, so that I am in despair" (69:20); and "The Lord is near to the broken-hearted, and saves the crushed in spirit" (34:18). It may be firm and steady: "My heart is steadfast, O God, my heart is steadfast" (57:7). Yet it may also be faint or erratic: "From the end of the earth I call to thee, when my heart is faint" (61:2): and "My heart throbs, my strength fails me" (38:10). The heart may be restrictive, closed, and unreceptive: "They close their hearts to pity; with their mouths they speak arrogantly" (17:10); and "So I gave them over to their stubborn hearts, to follow their own counsels" (81:12). Yet it may also be open, deep, and full: "My heart overflows with a goodly theme" (45:1); and "In him my heart trusts; so I am helped, and my heart exults" (28:7). The heart is also anxious and distressed: "My heart is in anguish within me, the terrors of death have fallen upon me" (55:4); and "I am utterly spent and crushed; I groan because of the tumult of my heart" (38:8); or "I was dumb and silent. I held my peace to no avail; my distress grew worse, my heart became hot within me" (39:2); or "My spirit faints within me; my heart within me is appalled" (143:4).

Because the heart may be identified with so many features of the self–emotions, intentions, desires, discernments–it follows that God's concern for the individual would be focused on the individual's heart. In Psalms, God is credited with knowing the deep secrets of the heart (44:21) and is portrayed as searching the heart to discover whether there are any evil intentions within it (17:3; 33:15; 139:23). Yet, God is more than the knower of hearts, for God is also, and more importantly, the one who regenerates the heart and restores it to its former health: "O Lord, thou wilt hear the desire of the meek; thou wilt strengthen their heart" (10:17); and "Create in me a clean heart, O God, and put a new and right spirit within me" (51:10); or "You who seek God, let your hearts revive" (69:32). Furthermore, God has a heart, and, as with humans, God's heart is the locus of discernment: "The counsel of the Lord stands for ever, the thoughts of his heart to all generations" (33:11); and "With upright heart he tended them, and guided them with skillful hand" (78:72).

In Psalms, the human heart is strongly associated with active seeking of God's help and assistance. One may call upon God with one's voice, but the voice is merely the heart's mouthpiece, and sometimes the heart experiences desires and emotions that are too deep for words. Thus, psalms talk about the need to pour out one's heart to God (62:8), to call upon God when one's heart is faint (61:2), and to entreat God's favor with all one's heart (119:58). Undergirding these prayers is a deep sense of trust that God will "incline" his own heart to the petitioners (34:18), even as they "incline" their hearts to God (119:36). The imagery here is of bending near, of bowing one's head and placing one's ear against the other's heart so as to hear its rhythms.

There is also a faint suggestion in the Psalms that if, through God's intervention, the heart can be revived, then perhaps the heart may go on forever: "The afflicted shall eat and be satisfied; those who seek him shall praise the Lord! May your hearts live forever!" (22:26). The flesh will surely die, but perhaps the heart–transplanted–will survive in some other place. If anything survives, it is the heart, the very center of the human self, the core of our sense of being an "I." Thus, at a time when the theological community is inveighing against the "I" because it associates the "I" with egoism (Nelson, 1989; Gelpi, 1989), the psalms not only affirm the "I" but give provisional thought to its immortality, basing this hope on evidence that, through God, the heart may be revitalized, restored to its former strong and rhythmic beating. It all depends, however, on the heart finding a hospitable home, and where else would this be but in the heart of God, so great and deep that it is capable of holding all human hearts in its remembrance?

This hope for the heart's transplantation into the heart of God is daring and risky, and goes against all conventional wisdom. It contrasts with Job's response to Bildad, one of his counselors, that unlike plants, humans have no prospect of coming back to life in another time or place. Bildad has just alluded to the plant whose roots "twine about the stone heap, living within the rocks," noting that if the rocks fail it, and it is destroyed, it will reappear elsewhere in the garden: "Behold, this is the joy of his way; and out of the earth others will spring" (8:16-19). Job agrees with Bildad as far as plants are concerned: "For there is hope for a tree, if it be cut down, that it will sprout again, and that its shoots will not cease" (14:7). But humans are different: "But man dies, and is laid low; man breathes his last, and where is he? As waters fail from a lake, and a river washes away and dries up, so man lies down and rises not again" (14:10-12). Thus humans are not like planted things, which are capable of living where they have been transplanted, but are like a dried up river which cannot replenish itself.

And yet, even in the midst of his lament over the eventual fate of the human self, Job allows himself to imagine another scenario in which God remembers him in the vale of death: "Oh that thou wouldest hide me in Sheol, that thou wouldest conceal me until thy wrath be past, that thou wouldest appoint me a set time, and remember me!" (14:13). Job does not say anything here about the heart of God, but God's heart is implied in his plea that God might set a time to remember him, as the heart–both God's and ours–is, above all else, the locus of memory and remembrance. The brain, porous and fickle, is notorious for its forgetfulness, while the heart, deep and steadfast, is known for its capacity to remember. As Luke says of Mary, Jesus's mother, she "kept all these things, pondering them in her heart" (2:19). This means, of course, that the heart may succumb to bitterness, nursing grudges, resentments, and hurts after the pain inflicted by another has long since subsided. Yet it also means that the heart may always find within itself grounds for hope, as it remembers times and circumstances when God heard its audible cries and its sighs too deep for words: "The Lord is my strength and my shield; in him my heart trusts" (Psalm 28:7).

PASTOR OF THE DISCERNING HEART

As hospital chaplains can readily attest, ministering to the potential recipient of a transplanted organ and to this person's family requires a discerning heart. Given the great risks that are often involved in organ transplants, and the distinct possibility that the body may reject another person's organ, there is the ever-present danger that hopes will be kindled only to be dashed as the body proves an unhospitable host to what it takes to be an alien intruder. The chaplain is caught in the classic bind of sharing the patient and patient's family's hopefulness while also anticipating that, sooner or later, these hopes may well be crushed. Even if the body receives the organ as a friendly guest, it is unlikely that the recipient or the family will ever be free from anxiety. Moreover, organ transplants tend only to extend life; they do not secure immortality, which, as we have seen, rests with God alone.

Yet, these very vicissitudes and ambiguities that surround the transplantation scenario underscore the profundity of the psalmists' view of human life as transient. In the psalmists' view, the transience of human life is perhaps its most self-evident feature:

> I have seen a wicked man overbearing,
> and towering like a cedar of Lebanon.
> Again I passed by, and, lo, he was no more;
> though I sought him, he could not be found.

> (Psalm 37:35-36)

If this psalm seems to suggest that it is the wicked who are especially transient, this would be misleading, for transiency is the fate of all people, regardless of whether their hearts are pure and clean, or deceitful and duplicitous. We are all like a leaning wall or a tottering fence, about to be brought down (62:3), and we are all like grass that flourishes in the morning and fades and withers by evening (90:5-6).

Mindful of human transiency, the psalms do not discourage us from entertaining the desires of our hearts–including the chance to live a fruitful life which has been extended by the surgical procedure of an organ transplant–yet, at the same time, the psalms caution against an overweening sense of personal grandiosity which causes one to believe that one's own survival is the most important thing in the world, and that sheer longevity is the key to a meaningful life. A psalm which captures this more circumspect view of one's personal existence is Psalm 131, which I quote in full:

O Lord, my heart is not lifted up,
my eyes are not raised too high;
I do not occupy myself with things
too great and too marvelous for me.
But I have calmed and quieted my soul,
like a child quieted at its mother's breast;
like a child that is quieted is my soul.
O Israel, hope in the Lord
from this time forth and for evermore.

Regarding our transiency, this psalm expresses a spirit not of resignation or passive acceptance, but of equanimity and inner peace. The vital image here is of a child who is held near its mother's heart. As the child listens to her heart's rhythmic beating, it is soothed and comforted.

Hope is not a friend of grandiosity but of modesty. It is uncomfortable around those who occupy themselves with things too great and too marvelous for them, but gladly communes with those whose hearts discern what is good and right for them. The chaplain or other pastoral care provider should have no difficulty encouraging hopes that derive from discerning hearts, and is often an active participant in the patient's and family's prayers–whether verbalized or not–for such discernment. Great skill is required of surgeons who remove and replace our vital organs. But no less skill is found among those who help a patient and family decide whether or not to undergo an organ transplant. This is not primarily a matter of ethics–however important ethical considerations may be–but is itself a matter of the heart. As Psalm 77 puts it: "I consider the days of old. I remember the years long ago. I commune with my heart in the night; I meditate and search my spirit" (vs. 5-6). And the familiar prayer of 19:14: "Let the words of my mouth, *and the meditation of my heart,* be acceptable in thy sight, O Lord, my rock and my redeemer."

PASTOR OF THE REGENERATED HEART

If the chaplain or other pastoral care provider is an instrument of hope through participation in the process of discernment, so is he or she a representative of the hope that, in God, the heart of an individual lives forever. As Selzer points out, the liver has great self-regenerative powers. Speaking of the effects of alcohol on the liver, he notes that the liver will

> grow back, regenerate, reappear, regain all of its efficiency and know-how. All it requires is quitting the booze, now and then. The ever-grateful, forgiving liver will respond joyously with a multitude of mitoses and cell divisions that will replace the sick tissues with spanking new nodules and lobules of functioning cells. This rejuvenation is carried on with the speed and alacrity of a starfish growing a new ray from the stump of the old. New channels are opened up, old ones dredged out, walls are straightened and roofs shored up. Soon the big house is humming with activity. (p. 76)

For the psalmists, the heart is also capable of being regenerated, and in much the same way, but such regeneration is the work of God. And because the heart can be regenerated, it is altogether appropriate for us to draw a certain parallel between the eventual fate of us humans and the plants of the earth. In lamenting his fate as a man who "comes forth like a flower, and withers," Job contrasts our fate with that of a tree which is seemingly indestructible:

> For there is hope for a tree,
> if it be cut down,
> that it will sprout again,
> and that its shoots will not cease.
> Though its root grow old in the earth,

and its stump die in the ground,
yet at the scent of water it will bud
and put forth branches like a young plant.

(Job 14:7-9)

What Job does not see–what he *cannot* see in his despair–is the fact that we have an organ beating inside of us which is remarkably similar to the tree that he describes, for it, too, is wonderfully resilient, and it, too, is often receptive to efforts to revitalize it, to bring it–quite literally–back to life. Unlike the ancient warrior who believed that the heart of another person, when ingested, would strengthen him, the chaplain or other pastoral care provider does not view the heart literally but metaphorically. This does not, however, mean that there is anything less real or true in his or her assurances that our hearts will live after our bodies have ceased to be. For with the Psalms, a crucial turning has already occurred from the literal to the metaphorical, so that it is possible for them to speak of those "in whose heart are the highways to Zion" (84:5).

THE PASTOR: INSTRUMENT OF HOPE

In emphasizing the role of the pastor in the process of discernment, and in offering assurance that God quickens the hearts of those whose lives on this earth have come to an end, I do not mean to overlook the other features of the heart, especially that it is the locus of emotions ranging from the heights of elation to the depths of despair. Nor do I mean to minimize the fact that the heart is a center of intentionality, and thus implicated in the moral task of deciding right from wrong, goodness from iniquity. But the specific issue which concerns us here–the pastoral care of the potential organ recipient and family–draws our attention specifically to the other features of the human heart: to the *desiring* heart (including the desire for longevity and even perhaps for physical immortality) and the *discerning* heart (which is concerned with attaining a deep sense of clarity and inner peace when faced with life's most difficult choices). It is in the tensions and ambiguities which inevitably emerge when the desiring heart and the discerning heart confront one another that hope itself is born. And the role of the chaplain and other pastoral care providers is, first and foremost, to be instruments of hope.

In standing thus at the crossroads of desire and discernment, the pastor's role as instrument of hope is not to encourage others simply to be "realistic" or to resign themselves to the non-realization of their heartfelt desires. As Proverbs suggests, hope is the ally, not the enemy of desire: "Hope deferred makes the heart sick, but a desire fulfilled is a tree of life" (13:12). So, as Paul W. Pruyser pointed out in an article published shortly before his death, where hoping is concerned, the issue is not whether a given desire is realistic,

> For anyone's grounds for hoping do not lie in the facts of reality, but in the ways in which reality has thus far disclosed itself to the person and in the meanings which that person has found in these disclosures. The fact that another person hopes where I would not hope indicates that his version of reality is different from mine. While seeing the point in my objections, if we were to argue with each other, he may still continue to hope and have his own grounds for doing so. (1986: 125)

Moreover, says Pruyser, concern with the meaning of reality involves more than an intellectual interest:

> It involves a passionate mental action, a choice, a commitment, in which one draws upon a philosophy of life, a religion, or an ethos that rings true to the tenor of one's experiences to date, and in some instances may be the fruit of a fresh insight newly gained from undergoing life-endangering or terminal illness. As a unique mental act or process, distinct among all forms of expecting, hoping allows a person in distress to assume that the universe is not wholly malign, that some benevolence is active somewhere; just as the hungry infant has come to assume from his experiences that his good mother not only feeds him but has herself the need to do so. (pp. 126-27)

Which brings us back to Mary, the mother of Jesus, who, in "pondering these things in her heart," revealed so much to us about the heart of discernment, and of how it not only gives to the desiring heart a new depth of understanding, but also provides grounds for genuine hope when the heart, accustomed to surviving on optimism, begins to faint or to break.

REFERENCES

Gelpi, Donald L., ed., 1989. *Beyond Individualism: Toward a Retrieval of Moral Discourse in America.* Notre Dame, Indiana: The University of Notre Dame Press.

Nelson, C. Ellis, 1989. *How Faith Matures.* Louisville, Kentucky: Westminster/John Knox Press.

Pruyser, Paul, W., 1986. "Maintaining hope in adversity." *Pastoral Psychology* 35 (2): 120-31.

Selzer, Richard, 1974. *Mortal Lessons: Notes on the Art of Surgery.* New York: Touchstone Books.

Theological Reflections on Organ Donation and Transplantation

M. Susan Nance, MDiv
William H. Davis, Jr., MDiv, ThM

> "I'm a walking-talking miracle," he declared with enthusiasm. "I was blind and dying, and now I'm alive and I can see!" The diabetic recipient of a pancreas and a cornea gave testimony to all who would listen as to how the Lord had blessed him so well and how he'd be a faithful witness to God's goodness and love for him. After leading us in a prayer of thanksgiving for his second chance and for those who in death had bequeathed to him an opportunity for new life, all the people said Amen.

The language of pastoral theology concerning the transplantation of organs has traditionally emphasized the experience of renewed life for the recipient. Persons are allowed to live again, perhaps to contribute significantly to the community if not their families. Surely, the reasoning suggests, the loving and merciful God who has

M. Susan Nance and William H. Davis, Jr. are Chaplain Supervisors at Duke University Medical Center, P.O. Box 3112, Durham, NC 27710.

[Haworth co-indexing entry note]: "Theological Reflections on Organ Donation and Transplantation." Nance, M. Susan, and William H. Davis, Jr. Co-published simultaneously in *Journal of Health Care Chaplaincy* (The Haworth Press, Inc.) Vol. 5, No. 1/2, 1993, pp. 137-144; and: *Organ Transplantation in Religious, Ethical and Social Context: No Room for Death* (ed. William R. DeLong) The Haworth Press, Inc., 1993, pp. 137-144. Multiple copies of this article/chapter may be purchased from The Haworth Document Delivery Center. Call 1-800-3-HAWORTH (1-800-342-9678) between 9:00-5:00 (EST) and ask for DOCUMENT DELIVERY CENTER.

© 1993 by The Haworth Press, Inc. All rights reserved.

guided us to this technology is pleased when men and women, once ill, are restored to health and wholeness.

> Herb* was near death when he finally received his new heart. He could easily remember, however, his life before the surgery. He spoke of sitting in his wheelchair with pencil-thin legs, too weak to walk or even feed himself at times. He cried watching his wife cut the grass and work the garden, for his yard had been his joy. The transplant gave renewal to his spirit and his body, each increase in the strength of his spindly calves giving rise to renewed faith and purpose in his life. He no longer felt the helpless observer: he was a "new creation."

The religious and/or spiritual support for individuals faced with the request for organ donation is also usually offered in the language of creation, redemption and reconciliation. Drawn primarily from Biblical perspectives, the notions of gift and new life are themes which pastors and chaplains may use with families in the shock and denial of early griefwork.

A theology of organ donation and transplantation which gives attention to the Genesis account affirms both the dignity and the responsibility of human beings for creation.[1] Life is a gift, and good. God, as author of life, entrusts the stewardship of the earth and its creatures to human beings. A gift of organ donation is therefore good stewardship because a brother or sister is given the opportunity to maintain or improve life. Organ donation is a sharing of God's resources with God's creation. Donation is also associated with the selfless act which may characterize the spiritual virtue of charity.

The donation of organs and tissue is also presented as a vehicle by which to give some good meaning to what may be an otherwise senseless tragedy.[2] A decision to donate becomes participation in affirming good over evil: Romans 8:28 becomes a way to claim hope in the midst of loss.

> It had been six months since her husband's death and Linda's grief was not without pain. She was able to speak with passion and emotion as a volunteer for the local procurement agency

---

* All names have been changed.

regarding her decision to donate his organs: "It helps me when I think that someone else lives even though I still miss Johnny very much."

Donation of organs may also suggest a continuation of life. For these families, death has not really taken place because the donor "lives on" through the living of the recipient(s).

Although the fact of successful organ and tissue donation has been in the public awareness for quite some time, and while most ecclesiastical authorities have formulated a theology of donation and transplantation, when pastoral care intersects with the moment of request for organ donation the response is still most often "no." It seems that the theology carried into the immediate donor situation, which is to say an impending or a recent death, is the donation theology of the pastor, not that of the grieving family.

The stewardship theology espoused by many people simply does not stand up in the crucible of asking the donation question. The practical theology of those who must respond to the question is one that begs for care rather than extends concern for others. Donation requests appeal to a level of generosity and stewardship which frequently seems unavailable to people caught in the pain of sudden grief–always the case in organ donation situations. What we do and how we feel at life's most critical moments is stronger than even our best intentions; our response may likely be, "I'm too needy to give right now." Like Mary and Martha responding to the death of Lazarus, in grief we may feel first and do theology second. What "feels" good for our grief pain is that which comforts and sometimes insulates, not necessarily that which fits our higher levels of theological reflection. A primary desire is for the pain to end, both the pain of the griever and the griever's perception of the suffering of the deceased: the loved one has suffered enough.[3] Another incision for an unknown patient, however needy, does little to ease the immediate trauma of loss and may exaggerate a sense of injustice.

Other than the wound in his chest and the massive amounts of his blood on soaked dressings and still pooling around the Emergency Room stretcher the young man looked healthy–the muscles of his arms, chest and legs gave testimony to his strength. It was a knife, wielded by a friend, they said, over a few bucks in a poker game that ended his life, the blade piercing the left ventricle of his heart. When his grieving mother was asked to give sight to some blind person through the donation of her son's corneas, it was too much pain to bear. She ran from the family room, her words testifying to her agony, "They cut out his heart and now they want to cut out his eyes."

The cornerstone of the pastoral care movement has been listening to and learning from the recipients of ministry for a better understanding of what people need. Conversations with bereaved persons point in several directions. The first aspect of the message from the recipients of our pastoral care is the primacy of emotion over intellect. In the case of the grieving mother we understand her need to give attention to her overwhelming pain and anger at the murder of her son. The gash in her heart needs our attention and the healing power of faith. And if we are to appeal to the hope that donation would in some way aid in her grief work, we must focus on her need before the needs of another.

We might help ourselves be better pastoral ministers if we remember that the grief wound is primarily a narcissistic wound calling for attention to the basic identity, self-understanding and spiritual awareness of the wounded. When we move to heal and comfort those in grief we encounter some who feel the incredible agony of Godforsakenness. In the absence of feeling God's presence it is not surprising that even the most faithful seek to hold on to all that they can and forbid any more taking apart of the loved one.

We need to rethink the attention we give to the basic split between human reason and human emotion that has us praising the power of redemption and healing evident in our successful transplant patients and yet railing against the use of our loved ones dead bodies. Most decisions made in the face of loss are emotional. We draw as much upon our horror at being dissected like some biology class frog as we do upon our fantasy of a new and disease-free life.

If organ donation holds the possibility of helping the donor with her/his grief, then our intervention on behalf of donation must relate to our efforts to comfort and care for the griever. Pastorally, this reminds of our need to be contextually sensitive, realizing that an emotional response may develop quite distinctly from an intellectual acceptance of the loss.[4] In many situations the chaplain or the pastor is the person who takes most responsibility for assisting the grieving family, and in those situations we need to remember that the family will face a decision about donation. The question about donation can become a part of the pastoral ministry to the family when it is posed with awareness of the particular grief process of that family. This ministry also necessitates the integration of the chaplain or pastor into the hospital team caring for the patient and the patient's family. All too often the question of donation is posed by someone who is external to the family's grief. Medical or other personnel who "pop the question" without knowing the emotional context of the family run the risk of galvanizing anti-donation bias, and we fail to serve the family in a way that makes donation a healing aspect of the grief process.

A second concern is for the for the "resurrection" of the physical body of the deceased, or for some, such as Jewish families, this issue may be voiced in terms of the "integrity" of the body after death.[5] Though some clergy may question the notion of such literal concerns for the "body" to remain together, the resolute hope of the bereaved is for a physical wholeness in the future. Clergy assisting families who are uncertain and who are seeking guidance may seek to clarify perceptions about the body. Genesis 3:19b, "Dust you are, to dust you shall return," (NEB), speaks to the understanding that the dead body does not remain intact until life is breathed into it again at resurrection day. Mortal bodies do return to dust. Christians might also consider the evidence that Jesus post-resurrection body was significantly different from his pre-death body.

Reflection upon any attempt of a pastoral care provider to "do theology" during the anguish of loss points to a third expressed need, that of facilitating better preparation for the event of the death of loved ones. Most church organizations have found the benefits of helping the faithful plan for giving through wills and living trusts. Can we focus the same intentionality towards the giving of organs and tissue? Infrequent worshipers as well as the most faithful members of our religious institutions turn to ministers for help in the face of grief, a not so silent reminder that grief is a profoundly spiritual experience. Preparation for inevitable future events would be one responsible way to assist individuals and families in making donor decisions. Conversely, negligence in exploring the option of donation may well eliminate the ability to choose.

We serve the needs of those who will face loss and those who wait for healing through donated organs when we make our places of worship and religious instruction forums for anticipating death and grief.[6] We may remind ourselves that all who benefited from the healing power of Jesus eventually died–at least physically. In addition, our preparation somehow needs to engage people emotionally as well as intellectually. We must affirm that the essence of our religious faith is spiritual truth, truth symbolized and lived out in our physical lives but not limited to our earthly, bodily existence.

Other concerns raised by patients and families add to our discomfort and may be too easily dismissed. Part of the difficulty is this: we as spiritual leaders assert seemingly opposing truths. On the one hand we affirm the truth of graceful stewardship in the donation of human organs and tissue, and, on the other, we affirm the freedom of individuals and families to deny use of their loved one's "parts" even for the most worthy of causes.

Some of these voices, the less privileged in our society, raise questions about the utilization of scarce resources. "If the technology and the finances were there for everyone who needed to get a heart or kidney or liver or pancreas, it might be different." Could it be that spending a hundred thousand dollars on one man's new heart might be better spent on prenatal care for hundreds or even thousands of impoverished, expectant, and often teenage mothers? Does the notion of stewardship not apply to the numbers of people who could be helped or healed with an effort equivalent to one person's healing through transplantation?

Another voice raised to the donation question has to do with our understanding of God and God's place as the sole divine creator, the being who gives life and takes it. When we, through medical technology including transplantation, grasp life victoriously from the jaws of imminent death, are we always acting within the divine will? Could it be possible that some people's reluctance to donate organs is related to the growing tendency in medicine to idolize our ability to sustain life at any cost?

Another theological chink is exposed when our notions of eternal life meet the practical extension of life for some donors.

> David's new heart was followed shortly by another gift. Although David never met the family of the young man whose heart he had been given, they, through procurement and hospital agencies, sent him their son's prized chess set. Since David now had the son's heart, the family reasoned he should also have something he loved. David's recovery was punctuated by visits to the hospital, and the chess set always came with him.

Does giving what had been a cherished piece of their son's life to someone who received his heart indicate a tendency to equate transplantation with immortality or even with resurrection? For David, the receiver of both the heart and the chess set, the gift was a constant reminder that he owed his life to someone else's death. The chess set seemed to play upon his conscience, making of his life a kind of game in which someone had to lose and forcing upon him the burden of winning.

As practical theologians we may need to live the tension between our pastoral voice and our prophetic stance in the face of medical technology that offers new and abundant life and also prolongs life as if medicine could save us from an ultimate death. Just as physical death was inevitably in the future for all who benefited from Jesus' healings, physical death is inevitable in all our futures. Longer life alone will not make us whole, even though it may offer us another chance for living out our hope.

NOTES

1. Thomisina, DC. The Quest for Organ Donors: A Theological Response. *Health Progress,* 1988; 69(7): 22-24.

2. Bartucci, MR. Organ Donation: A Study of the Donor Family Perspective. *Journal of Neuroscience Nursing* 1987; 19: 305-309.

3. DeLong, WR. Organ Donation and Hospital Chaplains. *Transplantation* 1990; 50(1): 26.

4. Coolican, MD. Katie's Legacy. *American Journal of Nursing* 1987; 87: 483-485.

5. DeLong, work cited.

6. Resources for clergy and community education are available in *Organ and Tissue Donation: A Reference Guide for Clergy* ($40.00) through South-Eastern Organ Procurement Foundation (1-800-KIDNEY-9) or United Network for Organ Sharing (1-800-24-DONOR).

Organ Transplantation and Tissue Donation: A Theological Look

O. Ray Fitzgerald, PhD

SUMMARY. The author's position is that the work of organ donation and transplantation and tissue donation over the past forty-five years is in need of theological reflection. Some profound events and processes are involved in transplantation as the human family engages in a quest for wholeness. Different religious traditions–Jewish, Catholic, Eastern Orthodox, and Protestant–view the use of organs for transplantation differently. General attribution theory is adapted as a perspective on organ transplantation.

Organ transplantation in human beings has a history of less than fifty years. It was only in 1947 that efforts of trying to utilize a donor kidney proved to be successful for a brief time. The year 1954 marked the first functioning human kidney transplantation in North America. In 1967 the world's attention was drawn to the first successful human heart transplant (South Africa). Also in the United States the first liver transplant was completed in 1967. The

O. Ray Fitzgerald is associated with the National Institutes of Health, Clinical Center, Bethesda, MD 20892.

[Haworth co-indexing entry note]: "Organ Transplantation and Tissue Donation: A Theological Look." Fitzgerald, O. Ray. Co-published simultaneously in *Journal of Health Care Chaplaincy* (The Haworth Press, Inc.) Vol. 5, No. 1/2, 1993, pp.145-160; and: *Organ Transplantation in Religious, Ethical and Social Context: No Room for Death* (ed. William R. DeLong) The Haworth Press, Inc., 1993, pp. 145-160. Multiple copies of this article/chapter may be purchased from The Haworth Document Delivery Center. Call 1-800-3-HAWORTH (1-800-342-9678) between 9:00-5:00 (EST) and ask for DOCUMENT DELIVERY CENTER.

© 1993 by The Haworth Press, Inc. All rights reserved.

development of the first tissue bank under the Naval Medical Research Institute, Bethesda, Maryland opened scientific doors which have greatly aided the transplantation endeavors.

In the past quarter century we have witnessed technology taking us through transplants of livers, hearts, lungs, and pancreas as well as cornea and numerous other body tissue exchanges. Further, the use of animal organs and tissues along with artificial means of carrying out human body functions have virtually exceeded human imagination. There are a number of theological questions and issues raised in these strides in human technology. The moral questions have real relevance as we explore what our Judeo-Christian responses are and need to be in the face of these challenges and opportunities.

My exploration of theological issues in organ transplant and tissue donations will be from Christian (Catholic, Orthodox, and Protestant) perspectives along with asking what responses also are coming from Judaism. Even though the literature carries serious writings about transplantation from countries like Japan and South Africa, for the most part our reflections will come in the main from North America. There are variations of responses and reflections which come from within both Christianity and Judaism. Our attention is drawn to scholars who write from a more generic perspective from within their respective traditions.

My theological, frequently enlightened by bioethical, reflections take me to serious inquiries. As a pastoral theologian, I seek the assistance of both classical and contemporary writings which will enlighten. The anticipated audience is persons like yourself who are interested in a theological perspective to guide you as you are either preparing for or providing services in the health care arena.

I am impressed that some of these serious inquiries are coming from persons as they are already seeking to reflect, while theological students, on how to apply theological principles to health care in the face of organ transplantation and tissue utilization. Two of these persons are Catherine (Cathie) Lyons whose reflections began in the 1960s while studying at the then Garrett (now Garrett-Evangelical) Theological Seminary[1] and Jeannette Clay Lucas who wrote her reflections in the mid 1980s while she was a student at Lexington Theological Seminary.[2] Cathie Lyons utilizes her own perspectives in the efforts of looking at world health needs as an executive with the United Methodist Board of Global Ministries in New York. Jeannette Lucas utilizes her perspectives as Hospice Director and Clinical Pastoral Supervisor in Lexington, Kentucky.

From the ivory towers of learning, Richard McCormick, S.J. as a theological/ethicist at Notre Dame University, John Meyendorff as theologian at the Orthodox Seminary of America, Martin Marty as church historian/ethicist at the University of Chicago and James Gustafson theologian/ethicist of Emory University, all have offered helpful perspectives for this writing. There is a necessary step back from the task of "doing theology" which takes much of the energy that many of us expend in hospital chaplaincies and in being a part of the physician-nurse-social worker health care team. Still another task is to reflect theologically on what our task means from a Judeo-Christian perspective.

CREATION AS CO-CREATORS WITH GOD

I believe it is useful to view our task of reflecting theologically from a perspective of Biblical Theology. My understanding is that what God created, as recorded in the narratives of the Hebrew scriptures, God called very good. Our perspective is that we are made in God's image. Creatures are on the earth to carry out the divine mandate in Genesis 1:28, "Be fruitful and multiply, and fill the earth and subdue it. . . ." (NRSV) We have come a long way from the "very good" of the Genesis record to our problems of human disease and earth pollution.

The interpretation of "subdue it" has been expanded to exploit, to pollute, and to stress oneself out by living out what the British poet wrote: "getting and spending we lay waste our powers." It seems the movement of the last half century has been that of seeking better ways to care for the human body and of necessity to begin asking what we are doing to planet earth. This is the context in which we are beginning to ask seriously how are we to be about our God's business in the world. Are we willing to view ourselves as co-creators with God?

One of the four principles which Jeannette Lucas uses for focus in her study is formulated as follows: "The Creator values what was created in the image of the Creator.''[3] In her perspective, "The Creator as manifested in human creation and human life is a projection of its Creator." This realization becomes profound in the realization that beyond being the projection of the Creator we can become co-creators with God.

When I was witnessing open heart surgeries first at the National Naval Medical Center in the late 1960s and later at the University of Kentucky Medical Center in the 1980s, I had a profound sense of this work being co-creation with God. Those of us who work in health care teams regularly can view this work as co-creation. Whether one is working as a profusionist, as a scrub nurse counting surgical sponges, or being the team leader in performing the surgery, each of these functions can be a profound kind of co-creation.

There continues to be a kind of mystery of what happens in the process of organ transplantation or other tissue exchanges. Since one of our pastoral learning methods is by case method, I want to share some reflections of a mid-1980s recipient of a heart transplant at Indiana Methodist Hospital in Indianapolis. Robert Clouse (his real name as reported in *Second Opinion)*[4] was and is a professor of history at a State University and pastor of a Church of the Brethren congregation.

Reverend Clouse/Professor Clouse follows an ideal model portrayed in the Gospels. When a healing took place he returned to thank those who were active participants in the drama. In Clouse's reflections this included (a) the donor family of a 30 year-old man in Buffalo, New York, (b) the surgical teams on both the giving and receiving end of the donated organ, (c) those who transported the heart by plane in a picnic cooler, and (d) his wife, Bonnidell, also a professor at the State University. Preceding all of these efforts were thousands of hours of research which were involved the refinement of the process. Also, in the earlier research work, hundreds of animals were sacrificed in the process.

Also there were various other necessary steps along the way. This includes both the surgical process and the accompanying necessary legislative steps which were needed for authorization. For example, I recall consulting with Kenneth Sell, MD, a medical researcher in the late 1960s. He was then a consultant to the Maryland legislature and now is Director of one of the eleven Institutes of the National

Institutes of Health in Bethesda, Maryland. As a Lutheran layperson, he was living out his discipleship by helping to define brain death and to support what became steps in federal legislation toward the development of the Anatomical Uniform Gift Act. These steps were in the foreground of Robert Clouse's receiving a transplant heart in Indianapolis two decades later. To be a co-creator means being active and engaged in the process.

In a normal developmental cycle humankind passes through stages of dependence and later independence to experience interdependence. We are to submit to a higher good as well as viewing the human family's work of subduing creation. Bernard Haring, a Catholic theologian, went beyond seeing the human task of salvation of one's own soul and preparing for the next world to include being a "co-creature of the future of many" as "a member of the redeemed human family."[5] Our awareness is raised by the realization that as health care team members we are moving toward experiencing interdependence in the transplantation in the process.

There is a desire to gain knowledge as one of the variations on the theme of co-creation. Persons may do this as scientists without an overt sense or acknowledgement that they are on "God's team." There are perspectives of local regionalisms about how both the human body and God's working in the world are viewed. It may be in the simplicity of religious faith expressed in America's Appalachian region or as the literalism which I experience now in the Mid-South and the Mississippi Delta region. Recipients of the transplants as well as their family and friends will bring their own religious perspective about the surgical and medical procedures and will tend to theologize about it. We have not done a very good job from our pulpits and classrooms to help either professionals in health care or the recipients of care to view God's active working in the process. It is more than a kind of fatalism which evokes passivity. As human beings we do have some control over our destiny.

THE RELIEF OF HUMAN SUFFERING

In scenes of persons turning an ashen color because of insufficient kidney functioning or gasping for breath because of limited circulation of the body's vital blood, the issue of suffering is highlighted. Suffering itself is as old as the human family. Anticipating the opportunity to relieve suffering draws many into health care professions. It became obvious that Robert Clouse, as cited above, and his family were suffering. In Judaism blood on the door posts meant suffering. In the Christian era the middle cross on Calvary as well as the crosses on the right and left meant suffering. Persons like both the Clouse family and the health care professionals need help in viewing the meaning of suffering.

There is a struggle going on two fronts around the issue of suffering. The medical community is making its response through the past forty-five years of both basic and applied science in health care. After forty years of efforts, which have turned out to be productive, the label of "Conundra Without End"[6] has been assigned. This issue confronts the medical community, moralists, and spiritual leaders alike. We are in an era of beeper medical calls, beeper ethics calls, and beeper spiritual guidance calls. In a modified message of the first telephone call we hear exclaimed: "What hath God (and medicine) wrought?"

To say the least, the genie is out of the bottle. The need has escalated for humankind to come to grips with the physical, psychic and spiritual suffering which is involved in the transplant process. Examples of where guidance is needed include more than 130 transplant centers in the United States alone. As well as having a goal of relief of suffering it is obvious that a lot of suffering is experienced by many persons along the way in the transplant process. Are we prepared to make appropriate responses to the question: "What is the meaning of suffering?" The scenes of Job are being relived—depressed, full of boils, and/or being misunderstood by friends and family.

A number of years ago I was actively involved in making a film entitled: "Beyond Medicine." The intention was to answer the question: "What does a Hospital Chaplain do?" I was then working closely with a Cardio-Thoracic Surgery Team. The team was led by Mitchell Mills, MD, now of George Washington University, Washington D.C. In the film I stated: "The question 'Why me?' or 'Why me and my family?' is the most frequently asked question in a Medical Center." It is entering into the arena of suffering with others which is called for especially from those of us who work from an acknowledged theological frame of reference.

Suffering deserves a response. Responses are at least three-fold. There is a medical response, a philosophical (ethical) response, and a theological/ethical (spiritual) response. There are somatic pains, psychic pains, and spiritual pains—each of which deserves a response. A genuine challenge is to have someone available when a person is seeking to plumb the depths of the meaning of his/her suffering.

The rhetorical question, "Why me?" is also an existential question. Some of us need to be willing and able to enter into the arena of human suffering. The person in distress wants some kind of response. A fully developed plan of spiritual care and psycho-social support will include the patient, the family, and the staff. There are some profound moments in the process of transplantation. There are times of spiritual awe and a sense of holy ground which helps us to link travail (suffering) as a stage along the way to desire outcomes of extended life and hopefully more meaningful life.

Let's take a look at some of the sufferings which deserve responses. Again, we use Robert Clouse as our case study. The donor family was hundreds of miles away from the Clouse family. They were in Buffalo, New York. We do not know the nature of the accident. Let us suppose that he (the later donor) was a married man and father of two children; he was hit by a drinking driver. Would it make any difference to us if he were the drinking driver or either the victim or perpetrator of the use of a hand gun? As this patient is dying, the family awaits word and hopes against hope. We wonder if some sort of spiritual and moral support is being given. In critical care waiting rooms interventions are important. These may be a willingness to listen to the unintelligible groanings and also the lashing out at God or others which becomes a part of the process. Persons are suffering; who hears and responds to the suffering?

Let's look at the team who has been called to "harvest" the heart and other organs and tissue. In their own projections team members such as a nurse or transplant coordinator, may see a spouse, a sibling, or a "significant other" in the dying victim. Who will be there to listen to these struggles? The impact of these experiences are best not left to chance. We need to become practical theologians in residence as well as to be expressors of empathy. To quote Anton

Boisen, a 20th century pioneer in the pastoral care movement, we need to help them make sense out of nonsense.

As an approach to the spiritual needs of the entire staff, Life Link, of (Tampa) Florida, has engaged the Reverend Albert Galloway as a full-time team member. Al's job is to be available to the staff, the families, and both donors and recipients of the donated organ. He began this kind of work a couple decades ago in Indianapolis at the Indiana University Medical Center and the Veteran's Administration Medical Center. In this sense he has become a theologian-in-residence, working on the team. Another key person is the Transplant Coordinator who extends services all along the psychosocial continuum. This person may also be asked questions which involve some profound theological reflections. A number of lay persons are finding new roles in interpreting the process from a spiritual dimension.

In following the Clouse family, who prepares the Reverend Clouse for his entry into the operating room? Who communicates to his spouse and children (sons then ages 20 and 26)? In my personal communication with Reverend Clouse, he stated that a Hospital Chaplain (Clinical Pastoral Education Intern) was with them. This person becomes priest, confessor, comforter and interpreter of the mysteries of God unfolding before the eyes of all who are a part of the process.

There is no final word on suffering in the organ transplant work. The attention I want to draw is to the spiritual and psychic suffering which is a part of the process. This can extend to the head of the surgery team especially when the morbidity rates go up. What is needed is a response from the community which takes into account the needs of the whole person. Wholistic/holistic care is needed to insure that body, mind, and spirit are cared for as part of one's entry into the health care arena. Part of the task of the pastoral care giver is to help with an interpretation of the meaning of suffering.

THE RESURRECTION AND TRANSPLANTS

Within the Christian tradition a belief in the resurrection has a very important place in coping with a crisis situation. Professor William F. May of Southern Methodist University offers an extended discussion about a belief in the resurrection as it relates to

organ transplants. He acknowledges that the body has some seven-
teen salvageable (transplantable) organs as well as useable tissue
including bone, skin, and nerves. My experience is that May errs on
the conservative side about traditional Christians who in his view
seem ". . . to forbid or discourage organ transplants."[7] In recent
studies nurses have been able to get a higher response to requests
for donations when they had come to grips with their own core
values on the matter. As well, other caregivers have to reflect on the
impact that is made on the family when survivors are approached
for a donation of organs and tissue.

However, I do think May raises a very valuable question: "Does
or should Christian belief in the resurrection of the body place
obstacles in the way of a new kind of removal from the body . . . ?"[8]
He makes a distinction between those who have difficulty with
cremation versus those who are willing to allow organs to be ex-
tracted from the donor. There are views of needing a whole body for
the resurrection which keep some people from being willing to be a
donor or keep their family members from being willing to sign for
organ or tissue donation.

What seems to prevail in both Christianity and Judaism is a
desire to show respect for the deceased. This can begin with a
request for a post-mortem examination. For the most part, Orthodox
Judaism does not approve of autopsies and this in part is a desire to
have the burial by sundown. What we are referring to is what the
late Professor Gordon Allport called sentiment. I recognize a need
to acknowledge how we do attach sentiment to memories of the
human body. It is the real world to deal with sentiments about the
body as we look at the person's belief about the resurrection. Here
is an area which calls both for discussion and a broadly based
educational response. Part of our task is to prepare and educate
people as to what their options are about stewardship of the body.
Rather than return these usable parts to nature, one option is to
recycle for use in extending life and well being of others.

PARALLELS BETWEEN THE EUCHARIST
AND ORGAN TRANSPLANTS

A very cornerstone of Christian teaching surrounds the place of
sacrifice. In the words of Jesus, ". . . No one has greater love than

this, to lay down one's life for one's friends" John 15:13 (NRSV). The Christian era was inaugurated by the sacrifice of Jesus. We are taught as we become a disciple we are to become available to persons in need. We give or offer some of ourselves as gifts or "living sacrifices" to others. This is highlighted in Luke's gospel in the telling of the stories of the Good Samaritan and of the Good Shepherd. The core theme of each story is the offering of either services or the totality of one's self to others in need. As we have God's gift for us in the Eucharist we can become bread and wine for our brothers and sisters in the human family.

In Eastern Orthodoxy there is a linking of a theology of the resurrection to a foundation for ethics. Professor John Meyendorff, the Academic Dean of St. Vladimir's Seminary in New York, does this in a writing on "Salvation in Orthodox Theology."[9] Salvation comes as we overcome in this life and anticipate the resurrection in the life to come. The church is the bearer of this good news of salvation.

THEOLOGICAL SIGNIFICANCE OF GENERAL ATTRIBUTION THEORY TO TRANSPLANTATION

I am proposing another way to view transplantation and tissue donation–from a phenomenological perspective. General attribution theory as articulated by Bernard Spilka of the University of Denver along with some other colleagues,[10] can be used to enable persons who are receiving organ transplants to put their own world view in perspective. I will elaborate on the three components of general attribution theory (1) Internal versus External Control, (2) Sense of Meaning and Purpose in Life, and (3) Sense of Self-Esteem. My thesis is that there is a theological dimension which needs to receive consideration. The question becomes: How is either recipient or donor viewing this process?

1. Internal versus External Control

For the sake of our discussion we will limit the question to only the organs of kidney or heart. One of the things we have learned is a person who has either chronic kidney or chronic heart disease feels very much out of control. Either body fluids are backing up or breathing is so labored and difficult that the person feels overcome by the deficiency.

Both organically and psychically, as well as spiritually, we are trying to help restore a sense of control. When one is on kidney dialysis or being sustained on a balloon pump for the heart, one feels very much out of control. There is a kind of helplessness and dependency which causes a person to experience regression. The utter dependence feeling is uncomfortable. In fact persons may feel themselves to be victims of technology or at least at the mercy of technology.

It is wholesome and healthy to attempt to help people regain a sense of internal control in their own lives. This concept presents parallels to a Christian perspective on conversion. Old things pass away giving way to the new. Receiving new/recycled organs is like becoming a new creation. One of the ongoing questions is: What meanings of these new experiences are being discovered by the recipient? Some would be uncomfortable calling a successful transplant a miracle. Certainly, even for the most fulfilled scientist who has experienced his/her hard work paying off, it does indeed remain a mystery. Perhaps this is one of the great psychic fueling processes as being a transplant team member—we are dealing in mystery.

One can view the transplant process as the drama of a priestly function at a holy altar where we see literally a human sacrifice being presented. This seems to be paralleled when we view the replacement of a body organ instead of retaining the diseased one. For many of us the Christian God accepts this sacrifice. One of the reasons I hold back viewing this precision work as a miracle is that sometimes there is a failure. There can be a rejection of tissue. The successes come when the new sacrifice (foreshadowed in the Eucharist) is accepted.

In salvific terms of need for a new organ we may begin asking: "Who sinned?" One response is that as we work with the human condition which involves freedom and choice we may still succumb to conditions and circumstances far beyond our control. Disease may potentially be a result of one's own gene pool which has become a given in life. Here is where grace (God's unmerited favor) is a part of the formula. It is a big step for any of us to let go of our control to One who gives us the freedom to work out our own destiny.

2. Sense of Meaning and Purpose

Phenomenologically and existentially a sense of meaning and purpose is a powerful concept. A person ponders the question dealing with the "why" of suffering (as stated above). A woman in travail about to deliver new birth certainly has asked this question. Either a man or woman who has experienced the terror and the threat of combat has asked this question. A patient who has experienced a vital organ malfunction has asked this question.

If there is any positive secondary gain which comes from human suffering caused by having diseased or otherwise malfunctioning organs, it is the opportunity to plumb the depths of the meaning and purpose question. Again, I'm brought back to the image of "holy ground." There is a sense that the struggle for health and wholeness becomes a morality play. We are involved in a process of listening as well as interpreting what is going on from an informed theological perspective.

The person who has experienced a chronic disorder has passed through stages inquiring into the meaning of suffering. Earlier in this writing I have addressed the "why" question. The meaning and purpose quest in life is a part of the "why" question. In following the story of Reverend Clouse with the heart transplant, he was asking what meaning and purpose is there for a 55 year old professional man with a diseased heart. In his case a Chaplain Intern became the theologian-in-residence to assist with the interpretation.

Religious systems thrive on persons who sense they have reached some point of extremity. Persons do not set out knowingly to create crises. They will happen. Those of us who commit ourselves to a theological perspective seek to equip ourselves and others with the means to deal with meaning and purpose questions. We may be able to help by offering some reflections when self talk has become counterproductive. A great part of this work involves story listening.

Over and over again in the past two decades we have dealt with the "quality of life" question. Artificial means of life support may have no way of promising quality of life. A few years ago we lived through the drama of both Barney Clark in Salt Lake City and William Shroeder in Louisville during their respective times of being kept alive by an "artificial heart." As we saw them tethered to a machine, the foreboding question of meaning and purpose overshadowed them. The theological task is to enable people to raise their own questions of ultimate concern and to receive an answer which is informed by a perspective of faith.

On any transplant team there is a need for a person who is prepared both professionally and personally to deal with the meaning and purpose question. Nature and destiny of humankind questions have been pondered by theologians as far back as the lay-theologian, David. He asked: ". . . what are human beings that you are mindful of them, mortals that you should care for them?" Psalms 8:4 (NRSV).

Out of the phenomena of working with persons experiencing grief due to the loss of friends or loved ones, we carry forth the idea of survivors guilt. For persons who receive a new heart, or as Bioethicist George Annas of Boston University refers to them as "recycled organs,"[11] it may be sometime before they overcome the self-talk and feelings that they are living because someone has died. My recommendation is for every transplant team as well as the donor team to have a "practical theologian in residence." I am experiencing a real need to see these persons better prepared to do these theological reflections.

My experience is that we have come a long way from the Cartesian body/mind split. We are attempting to deal wholistically with the spiritual dimension of the person. Even as I was preparing this article, I spent two weeks in Russia teaching and consulting on health care including the spiritual dimension of health care. My hosts kept reminding me that the Russian people are faced with a spiritual crisis. As President Boris Yeltsin prepared to come to America for consultation, he worshiped at a Russian Orthodox Church on the Eastern Pentecost Sunday (June 14, 1992). The reason President Yeltsin went to church and simultaneously announced that he was a "believing Christian," was that he was seeking "purification." This sounds like the heart and core of Judeo-Christianity. Without pushing the metaphor too far, it seems that a new form of democratic government was being transplanted and in the meantime there were reflex actions from the old.

One meaning and purpose which a person has, according to the late H. Richard Niebuhr, is to ". . . promote the increase of love of God and neighbor."[12] Health care crises which we are addressing in the transplantation issue offer considerable opportunities and a great challenge for theological reflection. Plumbing the depths of one's sense of meaning and purpose is a place to start.

3. Sense of Self-Esteem

The third dimension of general attribution theory focuses on the issue of self esteem. A paraphrase of this could be positive identity or sense of selfworth. In seeking a way of living out John 10:10, "I came in order that they might have life, life in all its fullness," (GNFMM) we are indeed looking for fullness of life.

A way of viewing life is from the aspect of right relationship. These relationships are three dimensional—past, present, and future. In dealing with the past the word reconciliation comes to mind. There was a time in certain American governmental hospitals that a patient was placed on lists, i.e., "Danger" or "Seriously Ill" or "Very Seriously Ill" list. This meant that the patient needed special attention about both temporal and spiritual matters. I am addressing, first, right relationships with self, others, and God as we view God.

I recall working in a large hospital with internal medicine patients. The perspective of one of the medical residents was stated well. When Doctor Charles Crummy summoned me as the On-Call Chaplain he said, "I've placed this patient on the 'Seriously Ill' list. Chaplain, it's time for you to help put the patient's spiritual house in order." We take initiatives in offering services as well as we reflect with the patients in their own concerns about relationships.

While working on a cardio-thoracic surgery team on a project which led to a doctoral dissertation, I began paying particular attention to pre-surgical preparation for open heart surgery patients. In pre-test/post-test measures, I discovered that appropriate attention to the inner spiritual world of the patient had very positive effects.

High self esteem enables a person to live more fully in the present. A positive outcome in organ transplantation gives a person more energy in the present. Some choose to view this experience as a gift from God.

They see that they have been given a second chance. In my contact with Reverend Clouse, the patient who has had the positive results with his six year old heart transplant, I became aware that he has seen very much what this second chance means. In my earlier work with heart patients, I concluded that a diseased heart may seem to produce in them a "sick self-image." Once health has improved there is a need for further work to help in the adjustment of what they are now able to do in terms of physical exertion and psychosocial functioning as these relate to change in self-image. There are good results in the shift to a positive change in self-image.

Persons who are enjoying "fullness of life" are able to see the future in both realistic and usually positive terms. For some a belief in immortality and the resurrection helps them to recall the Apostle Paul's words: "For me living is Christ and dying is gain" Philippians 1:21 (NRSV). They can now enjoy a new dimension of life.

General attribution theory enables people to put their own world view in perspective. In making a theological application to these new experiences we help interpret or at least reflect on the attributions persons are making to these experiences.

CONCLUSION

This paper set out to explore some theological issues in organ transplants and tissue donations. Early in the history of the transplantation process there appeared to be sparse reflections which made their way to theological and/or biomedical literature. The technology was developing faster than formal theological reflections were taking place. Protection of human subjects was a concern articulated by the presidential Commission for the Study of Ethical Problems in Medicine and Biomedical Research which convened in the 1970s.

When I surveyed a sample of the 130 Centers which do organ transplantation in the United States and also a sample of the renowned Bioethics Centers, I discovered that works are in progress on theological reflections, but they have not yet reached the public. One of these centers is the Parkridge Center in Chicago which published *Second Opinion* and commissions other serious works to be developed.

At a later time I will hope to bring an update on one of these efforts in the *Journal of Health Care Chaplaincy*. In the meantime I will welcome responses from others who know of works on theological reflection on organ transplantation which have not come to my attention.

REFERENCES

1. Lyons, Catherine. *Organ Transplants–The Moral Issues*, Philadelphia: The Westminister Press, 1970.

2. Lucas, Jeannette Clay. *Basic Moral Issues Involved in Transplantation and Related Theological Concerns*, Lexington, Kentucky: Lexington Theological Seminary (unpublished Master of Divinity thesis), 1986.

3. *Ibid.*, p. 8.

4. Clouse, Robert with Rodney Clapp, "A New Heart in the Face of Old Ethical Problems," *Second Opinion*, Vol. 12, pp. 13-24, 1989.

5. Haring, Bernard. *Medical Ethics*, Notre Dame, Indiana: Fides Publishers, 1973, p. 66.

6. Lyon, Jeff. "Coundra Without End," *Second Opinion*, Vol. 1, 1986, pp. 40-64.

7. May, William F. "Religious Justification for Donating Body Parts," *The Hastings Center Report*, February 1985, p. 41.

8. *Ibid.*, p. 41.

9. Meyendorff, John, "Salvation in Orthodox Theology," *Theological Studies*, 50, 1989, pp. 481-499.

10. Spilka, Bernard, Phillip Shaver and Lee A. Kirkpatrick, "A General Attribution Theory for the Psychology of Religion," *Journal for the Scientific Study of Religion,"* 1985, 24, (1), 1-20.

11. Annas, George J. "Feeling Good About Recycled Hearts," *Second Opinion*, Vol. 12, 1989, pp. 33-39.

12. Niebuhr, H. Richard. *The Purpose of the Church and Its Ministry*, New York: Harper & Press, 1956, p. 27.

About the Contributors

ARTHUR L. CAPLAN, Ph.D., is Director of the Center for Biomedical Ethics at the University of Minnesota. Dr. Caplan is author of numerous articles concerning ethics and health care. He is an internationally known ethicist and has long been interested in ethical aspects of transplantation. Dr. Caplan is also author of *If I Were a Rich Man Could I Buy a Pancreas and Other Essays on Medical Ethics,* Indiana University Press, 1992.

DONALD E. CAPPS, Ph.D., is William Harte Felmeth Professor of Pastoral Theology at Princeton Theological Seminary, in Princeton, N.J. Dr. Capps is author of several books on pastoral theology and numerous articles in pastoral care journals. His latest book is entitled, *Reframing,* Fortress Press, 1991.

MARILYN R. CLEAVINGER, M.S., is a biomedical engineer in the Artificial Heart Program at the University of Arizona Health Sciences Center. She has written extensively concerning artificial devices.

TERRY CONNOLLY, Ph.D., is a professor in the Department of Public Policy and Business Administration at the University of Arizona. He teaches courses in decision theory and has written many articles concerning the way decisions are made, both in healthcare and in other arenas.

JACK G. COPELAND, M.D., is the Michael Drummond Distinguished Professor of Cardiovascular and Thoracic Surgery and Chief of the Section for Cardio-Thoracic Surgery at the University of Arizona Health Sciences Center, in Tucson, Arizona. Dr. Copeland is a founding member of the *Journal of Heart and Lung Transplantation.* Dr. Copeland has written extensively concerning heart

© 1993 by The Haworth Press, Inc. All rights reserved. *161*

and lung transplantation and the use of mechanical assist devices for bridge to transplant procedures. Dr. Copeland has been leading the University of Arizona program since 1977.

WILLIAM H. DAVIS, Jr., M.Div., Th.M., is the Director of Pastoral Care and a CPE Supervisor at Duke University Medical Center in Durham, N.C. He is also president of Caring Eagle Associates, a consulting firm for growth and healing in organizations.

WILLIAM R. DeLONG, M.Div., is Chaplain at the University of Arizona Health Sciences Center, in Tucson, Arizona. He has been a member of the transplant program since 1988. Chaplain DeLong has published several articles about transplantation in medical and nursing journals, as well as in pastoral care literature. Rev. DeLong is on the editorial board of the *Journal of Health Care Chaplaincy* and the *Care Giver Journal* of the College of Chaplains.

O. RAY FITZGERALD, Ph.D., is a CPE supervisor and a certified pastoral counselor in Bethesda, MD. He is the editor of the *Journal of Health Care Chaplaincy*.

STACIE E. GELLER, M.A., is a graduate student in the Department of Public Policy and Business Administration at the University of Arizona. Her primary focus for research has been the way we make healthcare decisions.

M. THERESE LYSAUGHT, Ph.D., is Associate for Religion, Culture, and Health Care Ethics at the Park Ridge Center for the Study of Health, Faith and Ethics, in Chicago, IL. Dr. Lysaught has published on widely different topics concerning ethics, theology and health care. Her current interests include transplantation, physician-assisted suicide, notions of normalcy and genetic engineering. Before coming to the Park Ridge Center, Dr. Lysaught taught ethics at Duke University.

DEBORAH MATHIEU, Ph.D., is an assistant professor in the Department of Political Science at the University of Arizona. She has written several books including, *Organ Replacement Technology.* Dr. Mathieu is on the ethics committee at University Medical Center, and teaches graduate and undergraduate classes in medical ethics.

ANNE NICHOLSON MACDONALD, R.N., M.S., is a transplant coordinator with the University of Arizona's Department of Cardiovascular and Thoracic Surgery since 1985. She has published several articles concerning various aspects of transplantation and co-authors a chapter on heart transplantation in *Tissue and Organ Transplantation: Implications for Professional Nursing Practice,* ed. S. Smith, C.V. Mosby, 1990.

JEREMIAH J. McCARTHY, Ph.D., is a catholic priest and Dean of St. John's Seminary in Camarillo, CA. Rev. McCarthy teaches medical ethics and lectures on the catholic perspective of many issues relating to health care. He is co-author of *Medical Ethics: A Catholic Guide to Health Care Decisions,* Liguori Publications, 1990.

M. SUSAN NANCE, M.Div, is a chaplain and CPE Supervisor at Duke University Medical Center in Durham, N.C. She is a Southern Baptist minister and has been with the Department of Pastoral Care at Duke since 1988.

RICHARD G. SMITH, M.A., is a biomedical engineer in the Artificial Heart Program at the University of Arizona Health Sciences Center. He has written extensively concerning artificial devices.

TIM THORSTENSON, M.Div., is a CPE Supervisor with the Department of Pastoral Care at Abbott Northwestern Hospital in Minneapolis, MN. Rev. Thorstenson has been chaplain with the Cardio-Thoracic Replacement Program at Abbott since 1986.